DRESSING LONG HAIR

Published by Patrick Cameron Hair International

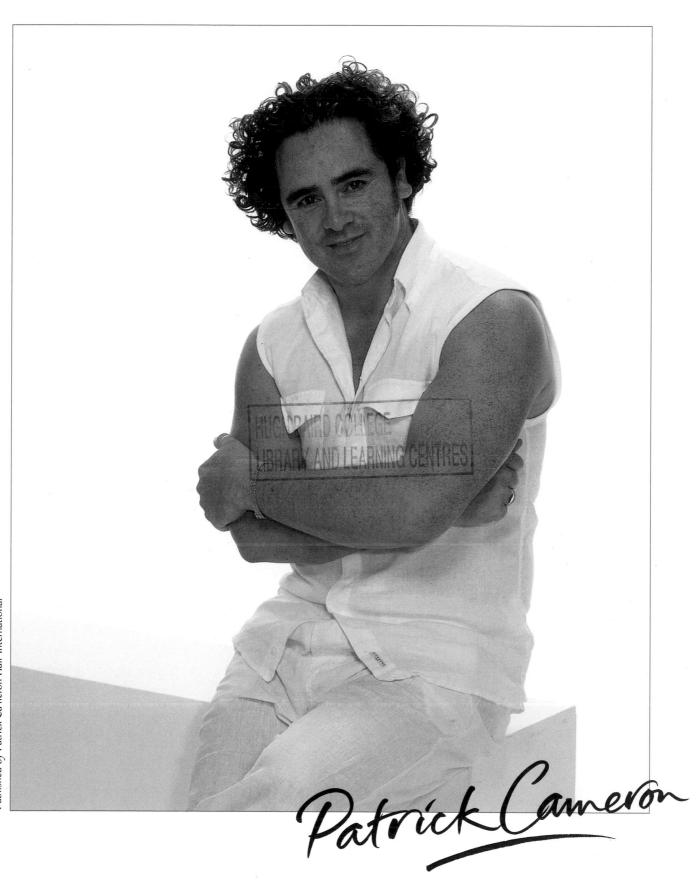

Patrick Cameron

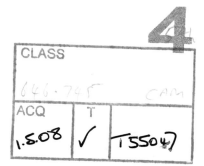

CONTENTS

Dear reader,

I am delighted to be able to present you with my third step by step long hairdressing book. I am often surprised to hear people tell me that they are frightened of working with long hair. Experience has shown me that if you approach long hairdressing simply and methodically, step by step, just the same way that you learned to cut hair then the results will speak for themselves. 'Dressing Long Hair Book 3' is a way to further your confidence, through knowledge and training and hopefully give you some new ideas that will serve you well for the rest of your career.

This book and my other educational vehicles are really just guidelines for the hairdresser to follow. Once you have mastered the basic techniques involved in creating a style it is up to you to place your own stamp of creativity and originality on your work. In my training school here in London and around the world I am constantly thrilled to see hairdressers using my ideas and techniques and making them their own. Sharing my methods in this way brings back ten fold reward in the way of new inspiration.

I hope that you enjoy this book as much as I have enjoyed putting it together.
15 styles, step by step ... go ahead ... have fun and create!!!!

Patrick Cameron

Patrick Cameron

Lieber Leser, liebe Leserin,

vor Ihnen liegt mein drittes Buch für das schrittweise Frisieren von langem Haar. Mich erstaunt es immer wieder, wenn ich höre, wie viele Friseure vor dem Frisieren von langem Haar zurückschrecken. Dabei müssen Sie nur methodisch Schritt für Schritt vorgehen, so, wie Sie das beim Haarschneiden gelernt haben. Glauben Sie mir, die Mühe lohnt sich! Das „Dressing Long Hair Book 3" gibt Ihnen das Selbstvertrauen und die Gewissheit, wie Sie mit Übung und Ausdauer Erfolg haben können, und zeigt Ihnen ein paar neue Ideen, von denen Sie hoffentlich während Ihrer gesamten beruflichen Karriere profitieren können.

Dieses Buch und meine anderen Lehrmaterialien sind im Grunde genommen nichts anderes als Anregungen für den Friseur. Sobald Sie die Grundtechnik für eine Frisur beherrschen, können Sie sie ganz nach Ihrem Geschmack abändern. Ich bin immer wieder aufs neue begeistert, wenn ich sehe, wie Friseure in meiner Friseurschule in London und weltweit aus meinen Ideen und Techniken neue machen. Weil meine Methoden anderen als Anregung dienen sollen, werde ich um das Zehnfache belohnt.

Ich hoffe, dass Ihnen die Lektüre dieses Buches genauso viel Freude bereitet wie mir das Zusammenstellen.
15 Frisuren, Schritt für Schritt ... Fun und Kreativität sind keine Grenzen gesetzt!!!!

Patrick Cameron

Patrick Cameron

Caro lettore

Sono lieto di presentarle il mio terzo libro per acconciature raccolte con semplici istruzioni a passaggi. L'esperienza mi ha dimostrato che se applichiamo un metodo razionale per realizzare una acconciatura raccolta, a passaggi, come nella esecuzione di un taglio, avremo dei risultati sorprendenti. Dressing Long Hair Book 3 e' un modo per migliorare la sua fiducia nelle sue abilita' e per darle nuove idee che le saranno utili per il resto della sua carriera.

Questo libro insieme con i miei altri supporti didattici sono solo una linea guida per imparare le tecniche di base e per stimolare la sua creativita' e originalita' nella realizzazione delle acconciature raccolte. Nella mia scuola di acconciatura a Londra non smette mai di sorprendermi l'interpretazione dei miei look dagli studenti. Condividere le mie idee mi ricompensa e contribuisce tantissimo alla formazione di nuove idee.

Mi auguro che si diverta a realizzare queste acconciature quanto e' stato divertente per me crearle. 15 look con semplici passaggi...coraggio...si diverta e crei!!!

Patrick Cameron

Patrick Cameron

Cher lecteur,

Je suis ravi de pouvoir vous présenter mon troisième livre de procédures détaillées de coiffure pour cheveux longs. Je suis souvent surpris d'entendre les gens me dire qu'ils ont peur de travailler sur des cheveux très longs. L'expérience m'a appris que si l'on aborde la coiffure des cheveux longs de façon simple et méthodique, une étape après l'autre, de la même manière que l'on apprend à couper les cheveux, les résultats se passent de commentaires. Le troisième livre de coiffure des cheveux longs est destiné à vous donner confiance, en vous offrant connaissances et exercices pratiques et il vous fournira peut-être également quelques idées nouvelles qui vous serviront tout au long de votre carrière.

Ce livre, comme mes autres publications d'enseignement, ne contient que des principes généraux que les coiffeurs sont invités à suivre. Une fois qu'ils ont maîtrisé les techniques de base requises pour la création d'un style, ils sont libres de les développer avec créativité et originalité dans leur propre travail. Dans mon centre de formation ici à Londres et partout dans le monde, je ne cesse d'être enchanté par la manière dont les coiffeurs utilisent mes idées et mes techniques et les transforment pour se les approprier. Partager mes méthodes de cette manière me récompense plus de dix fois en me permettant de découvrir des formes d'inspiration nouvelle.

J'espère que ce livre vous apportera autant de plaisir que j'en ai eu à l'écrire.
15 styles, des descriptions détaillées... allez-y... amusez-vous et ajoutez vos propres créations !

Patrick Cameron

Patrick Cameron

Querido lector:

Tengo el placer de presentar mi tercer libro de peluquería paso a paso para cabellos largos. Cuando la gente me dice que les aterra trabajar con cabellos largos siempre me toma por sorpresa. La experiencia me ha enseñado que si se afronta el peinado de los cabellos largos de forma sencilla y metódica, paso a paso, del mismo modo que hemos aprendido a cortar el cabello, los resultados hablarán por sí mismos. El "Tercer Libro de Peluquería para Cabellos Largos" le ayudará a aumentar su confianza proporcionándole conocimientos y formación, y espero que le aporte nuevas ideas que le resulten de utilidad durante el resto de su trayectoria profesional.

Tanto este libro como mis otros vehículos educativos deben utilizarse solamente a modo de orientación para el peluquero. Una vez domine las técnicas básicas necesarias para crear un peinado, dependerá de usted dejar su sello personal con la creatividad y la originalidad de su trabajo. En mis escuelas, en Londres y en todo el mundo, siempre me encantar ver que los peluqueros utilizan mis técnicas y mis ideas y las convierten en las suyas propias. Compartir mis métodos de esta forma supone una gran recompensa que me ayuda a encontrar nuevas fuentes de inspiración.

Espero que disfrute de este libro tanto como yo he disfrutado recopilándolo. 15 peinados, paso a paso…. Adelante: ¡diviértase y dé rienda suelta a la creatividad!

Patrick Cameron

Patrick Cameron

読者の皆様へ

このたびは「ロングヘアのためのステップ・バイ・ステップ・ヘアドレッシング第三巻」を皆様にお届けすることができ大変うれしく思います。ロングヘアのヘアドレッシングは苦手という方が多くいらっしゃることに私はいつも驚きを感じます。私の経験ではロングヘアのドレッシングの成功の秘訣はカットの仕方を習ったときとまったく同様、ステップ・バイ・ステップにシンプルに系統立てたアプローチで学ぶことであると感じています。「ロングヘアのためのステップ・バイ・ステップ・ヘアドレッシング第三巻」では皆さんが理論と実践を通して、さらに自信をつけられるようになっており、また今後お仕事を続けられる上でおおいに役に立つ真新しいアイデアも発見していただけることと思います。

この本をはじめ、私が執筆の教材類はあくまでも美容師の皆さんにガイドラインとして参考にしていただくものです。いろいろなスタイルを作り上げるための基本的なテクニックを習得したらあとは皆さん次第です。ぜひ、ご自分の創造性と独創性を活かしてください。ここ、ロンドンや世界の私のトレーニングスクールで美容師の皆さんが私のアイデアやテクニックを学び、自分のものとされているの目にするのは私にとっては大きな楽しみです。また、新たなインスピレーションを与えてくれ、大きなやりがいを感じています。

私はおおいに楽しみながらこの本の執筆にあたりましたが、皆さんにもぜひ楽しくこの本を活用していただけることを望んでいます。
15種類のいろいろなスタイルを紹介しています。ステップ・バイ・ステップ、遊び感覚で挑戦してみてください。

Patrick Cameron

パトリック・キャメロン

亲爱的读者，

我很高兴能向您展示我的第三本长发发饰入门。我经常吃惊讶地听到有人跟我说他们对长头发不知所措。经验告诉我：如果您一步一步地处理长发发式简单而有条理，就像您学习剪发的方法，那么结果是不言自喻的。"长发发饰3"是通过知识和训练，给您新的想法，进一步增长您的自信，为您今后的工作服务。

此书以及本人的其他教育工具的确是美发师遵循的指南。一旦您掌握了塑造发型的基本技巧，就可以在工作中自由发挥创造。这里的以及我世界各地的培训学校里，我不断激动地看到美发师运用我的主意和技巧，也创造他们自己的东西。以此享用我的方法，新的灵感层出不穷。

我喜欢编写此书，也希望您喜欢这本书。
十五款发饰，一步一步向前，享受并创新！！！

Patrick Cameron

帕奇克·卡迈龙（Patrick Cameron）

سيدي العزيز/سيدتي العزيزة،

يسرني أن أقدم إليكم كتابي الثالث الذي يفصّل إجراءات تسريح وتزيين الشعر الطويل.

مراراً ما أندهش عندما أسمع الناس يقولون لي أنهم يتخوفون من تصفيف الشعر الطويل. ولكن الخبرة علمتني أنكم إذا تعاملتم مع تسريح الشعر الطويل ببساطة ومنهج منتظم، خطوة بعد خطوة، تماماً مثلما تم على قص الشعر، فلا بد أن يتحقق لكم النجاح المنشود. وهذا الكتاب «تصفيف الشعر الطويل المجلد ٣» يساعدكم على تعزيز ثقتكم في العمل من خلال زيادة المعرفة والتدريب، كما أأمل أن يعطيكم بعض الأفكار الجديدة تستفيدون منها على ممر الزمن.

إن هذا الكتاب مع مطبوعاتي التعليمية الأخرى هو عبارة عن إرشادات عامة موجهة الى مزين الشعر. فبعد أن تتقن الأساليب الأساسية المستخدمة في خلق تسريحة شعر معينة يبقى عليك إضافة اللمسات النهائية من إبداعك وإبتكارك. إنه من دواعي سروري وفرحي أن أرى في مدرستي هنا في لندن وفي مراكز التدريب الأخرى حول العالم التابعة لي مزيني الشعر يستخدمون أفكاري وأساليبي ويوالفونها حسب طرازهم الشخصي. ومشاركة خبرتي وأساليبي في العمل بهذه الطريقة يكافئني مضاعفاً كما ويحفزني على إستباط وإستلهام أفكار وآراء جديدة.

إنني آمل أن تستمتعوا بهذا الكتاب كما إستمتعت أنا في تأليفه وجمعه.

إليكم ١٥ تسريحة مفصلة خطوة فهيّا بكم – جربوها وتمتعوا بممارستها مع إضافة ما لديكم من لمسات شخصية.

Patrick Cameron

باتريك كاميرون

WHITE LADY

• Section from nape to crown 2cm wide (fig. 2) • Twist middle section tightly, piece by piece to create base (fig. 3-7) • Brush a section from the side over base, twist and pin under base. Repeat left to right (fig. 9-16) • Tie tails into knots over pinned areas (fig. 18-21) • Split top section in two. Twist back and pin (fig. 22-24) • Spray and place top hair tails softly (fig. 25-26)

• Vom Nacken bis zum Scheitel eine 2 cm breite Haarsträhne abtrennen (Abb. 2) • Den Mittelbereich Stück für Stück fest verdrehen, um das Unterhaar zu bilden (Abb. 3-7) • Einen Haarabschnitt von der Seite über das Unterhaar bürsten, verdrehen und unter dem Unterhaar feststecken. Abwechselnd links und rechts wiederholen (Abb. 9-16) • Die Strähnen über den festgesteckten Haarabschnitten verknoten (Abb. 18-21) • Das Oberhaar zweiteilen. nach hinten bürsten und feststecken (Abb. 22-24) • Haarspray aufsprühen und die oberen Strähnen weich verteilen (Abb. 25-26)

• Separare una sezione di 2cm dalla nuca alla sommita' del capo (figura 2) • strettamente la sezione centrale un poco alla volta per creare la base (figure 3-7) • Spazzolare una sezione dal lato, sopra la base e fermare sotto la base. Ripetere i passaggi da sinistra a destra (figure 9-16) • Formare dei nodi sopra la base (figure 18-21) • Dividere la parte superiore in due. Attorcigliare e fermare (figure 22-24) • Spruzzare e disporre le ciocche nella maniera desiderata (figure 25-26)

• Séparez une section large de 2 cm de la nuque en haut de la tête (fig. 2) • Enroulez de manière serrée la section du milieu, morceau par morceau, pour créer une base (fig. 3-7) • Brossez une section latérale sur la base, enroulez et épinglez sous la base. Répétez la procédure de gauche à droite (fig. 9-16) • Attachez les tresses en nœuds sur les sections épinglées (fig. 18-21) • Divisez en deux la section supérieure. Enroulez vers l'arrière et épinglez (fig. 22-24) • Vaporisez et placez doucement les tresses supérieures (fig. 25-26)

• Separar una sección desde la nuca hasta la coronilla de 2 cm de ancho. (Fig. 2) • Enrollar la parte central de forma que quede bien apretada, pieza por pieza, para crear la base. (Fig. 3-7) • Cepillar una sección de los laterales sobre la base, enrollar y sujetar bajo la base. Repetir de izquierda a derecha. (Fig. 9-16) • Atar las coletas en forma de nudos en las zonas sujetas con clips. (Fig. 18-21) • Dividir la sección superior en dos partes. Enrollar hacia atrás y sujetar con un clip. (Fig. 22-24) • Aplicar laca y distribuir las coletas superiores con cuidado. (Fig. 25-26)

• えりあしからクラウンにかけて、幅2cmのセクションをとる。(図2) • 中央のセクションを部分ごとにとり、きつくツイストしてベースを作る。(図3-7) • ベースの上にかけてサイドからセクションをブラッシングし、ツイストしてベースの下にピンに留める。左から右へ繰り返す。(図9-16) • ピンで留た箇所の上でテールを作り結ぶ。(図18-21) • トップを二つに分ける。後部へツイストし、ピンで留める。(図22-24) • トップヘアのテールをスプレーし、そっとおく。(図25-26)

• 从后颈到头顶头发2厘米宽（图2） • 中间头发一片一片编织紧密，形成发基（图3-7） • 从旁梳一片头发，编结夹在发髻基下面。从左到右重复（图9-16） • 在夹发处上边发梢结（图18-21） • 头顶头发分两片。向后编结，发卡夹住（图22-24） • 喷发胶，轻轻地摆设头部发梢（图25-26）

• قسّم الشعر الى خُصل إبتداء من قفا العنق الى ذروة الرأس بعرض ٢ سم للخصلة الواحدة (الصورة ٢) • إفتل الخصلة الوسطى بشدة على مقاطع، الواحد بعد الآخر لتكوين القاعدة (الصور ٣ الى ٧) • سرّح خصل الشعر واحدة بعد الأخرى بالفرشاة من جهة اليمين للقاعدة وضعها فوق القاعدة ثم ثبتها بدبابيس تحت القاعدة. كرر هذا الإجراء من اليسار الى اليمين (الصور ٩ الى ١٦). • أربط ذيول الخصل في عقد فوق مواضع التثبيت بالدبابيس لتغطيتها (الصور ١٨ الى ٢١) • أفصل القسم الأمامي من الخصلة الوسطى الى شطرين ثم إفتل كل خصلة منها نحو الوراء وثبتها بدبابيس. (الصور ٢٢ الى ٢٤) • رش التسريحة وإضبط ذيول الشعر العليا بلطف (الصورتين ٢٥ الى ٢٦)

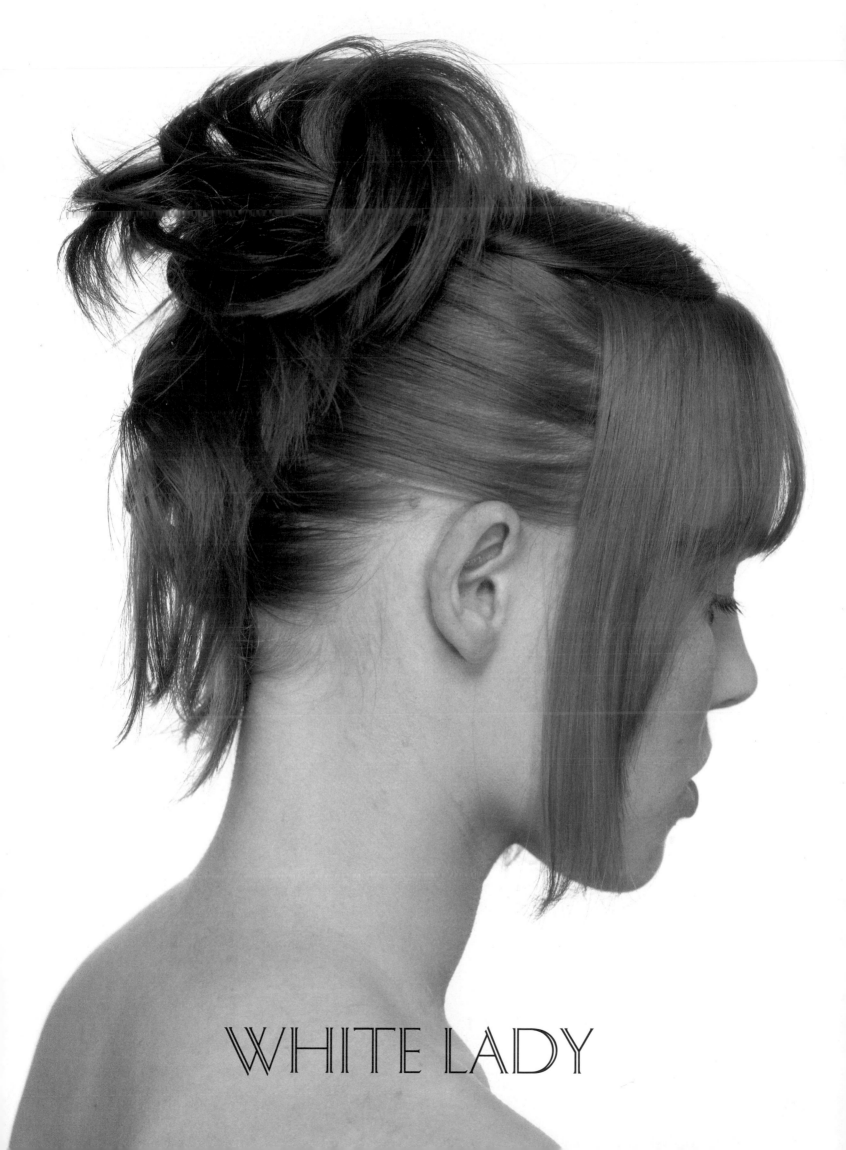

WHITE LADY

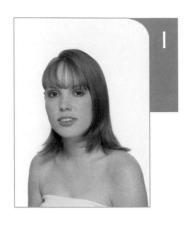

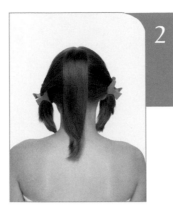

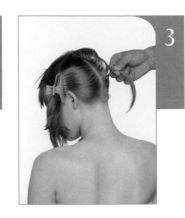

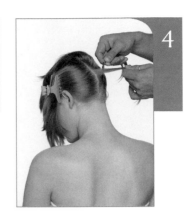

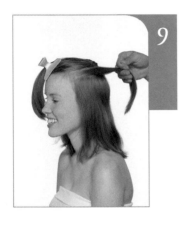

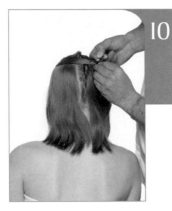

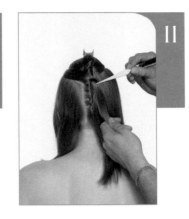

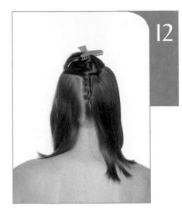

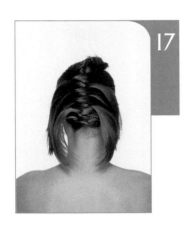

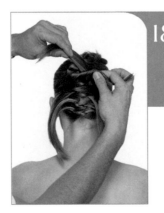

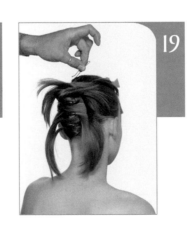

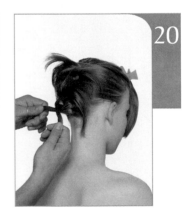

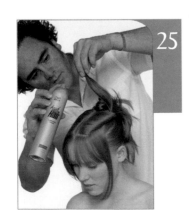

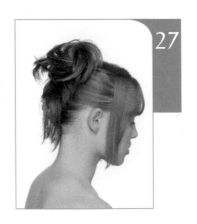

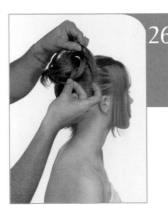

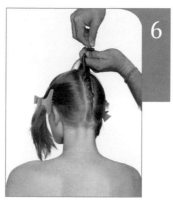

5

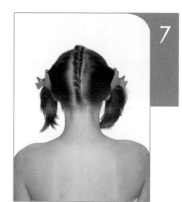

6

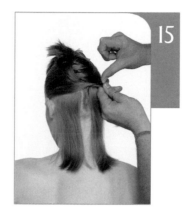

7

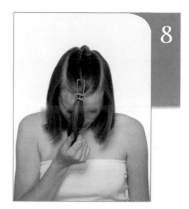

8

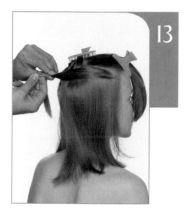

13

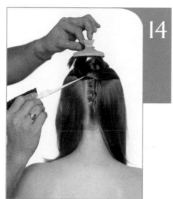

14

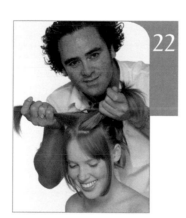

15

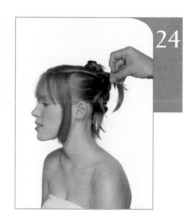

16

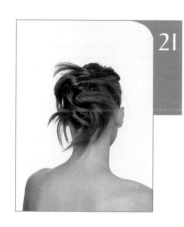

21

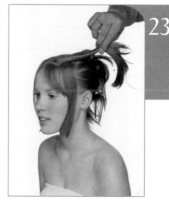

22

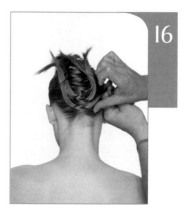

23

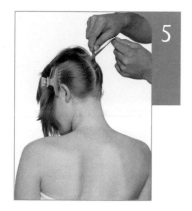

24

WHITE WEDDING

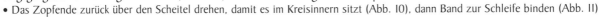

• Slice a section from front to behind crown and place into ponytail. (fig. 2) • Tie ribbon to base (fig. 3) • Twist ponytail towards the face and twist ribbon opposite way (fig. 4) • Add another section by taking hair under and over twist. Repeat. (fig. 5-6) • Keep binding ribbon in opposite direction section by section (fig. 7-8) • Pin end of twist into ponytail base (fig. 9) • Place tail of twist back over crown to sit inside circle (fig. 10) tie ribbon into bow (fig. 11)

• Einen vorderen Haarabschnitt hinter dem Scheitel zu einem Pferdeschwanz formen. (Abb. 2) • Band am Haaransatz festbinden (Abb. 3) • Den Pferdeschwanz zum Gesicht hin drehen und das Band in entgegengesetzte Richtung drehen (Abb. 4) • Einen anderen Haarabschnitt hinzunehmen und das Haar abwechselnd über und unter den gedrehten Zopf bringen. Wiederholen (Abb. 5-6) • Das Band Strähne um Strähne in die entgegengesetzte Richtung einflechten (Abb. 7-8) • Das Ende des gedrehten Zopfes am Ansatz des Pferdeschwanzes feststecken (Abb. 9) • Das Zopfende zurück über den Scheitel drehen, damit es im Kreisinnern sitzt (Abb. 10), dann Band zur Schleife binden (Abb. 11)

• Fate una coda prendendo una sezione dalla sommita' del capo (figura 2) • Legare un nastro alla base (figura 3) • Attorcigliare la coda in senso antiorario e attorcigliare il nastro nella direzione opposta (figura 4) • Aggiungere un'altra ciocca facendola passare da sotto e continuando ad attorcigliare, ripetendo il passaggio con ogni ciocca (figure 5-6) • Continuate ad avvolgere il nastro nella direzione opposta un poco alla volta (figure 7-8) • Fermate i capelli attorcigliati sulla base della coda (figura 9) Disporre i capelli rimasti all'interno del cerchio creato (figura 10) annodando il nastro (figura 11)

• Prenez une section allant du devant à l'arrière du haut de la tête et faites une queue de cheval. (fig. 2) • Attachez le ruban sur la base (fig. 3) • Enroulez la queue de cheval vers le visage et enroulez le ruban dans le sens opposé (fig. 4) • Ajoutez une autre section en prenant les cheveux par-dessous et en les enroulant. Répétez la procédure (fig. 5-6) • Continuez à attacher le ruban dans le sens opposé, section par section (fig. 7-8) • Epinglez l'extrémité de la spire dans la base de la queue de cheval (fig. 9) • Pliez l'extrémité de la spire sur le haut de la tête en forme de cercle (fig. 10), à savoir le ruban doit former un nœud (fig. 11)

• Separar una sección desde la parte superior hasta la parte posterior de la coronilla y hacer una cola. (Fig. 2) •Atar una cinta la base. (Fig. 3) • Enrollar la cola en dirección al rostro y enrollar la cinta en la dirección opuesta (Fig. 4) • Añadir otra sección, tomando el cabezo de la parte inferior y superior de la cola enrollada. Repetir la operación. (Fig. 5-6) • Seguir enrollando la cinta en la dirección opuesta, sección por sección. (Fig. 7-8) • Sujetar con un clip la punta de la parte enrollada en la base de la cola. (Fig. 9) • Colocar la punta de la parte enrollada sobre la corona de forma que quede dentro del círculo (Fig. 10) y atar la cinta con un lazo. (Fig. 11)

•クラウンの前から後ろへセクションをとり、ポニーテールを作る。（図2） •ベースにリボンを結ぶ。（図3） •顔の方向に向けてポニーテールをツイストし、リボンを反対側にツイストする。（図4） •ツイストの上と下からヘアをもってきて、次のセクションを作る。繰り返す。（図5-6） •セクションごとにリボンを反対の方向に縛りつけていく。（図7-8） •ポニーテール・ベースの中でツイストの終端をピンで留める。（図9） •ツイストのテールをクラウンの上にもってきて、円の形にする。（図10）リボンを蝶結びにする。（図11）

•从头顶前到头顶后选一片头发，扎成马尾。（图2） •在发根处扎发带(图3) •朝面部编结马尾，并发带向反方向编。（图4） •通过从编结的头发的上方和下方增加另一片头发。重复。（图5-6） •继续按反方向一片一片头发绑发带(图7-8) •把辫梢夹入马尾发根(图9) •将辫尾盘在头顶置于环中(图10)即发带成弓形(图11)

• أفصل خصلة من المقدمة الى ما وراء ذروة الرأس بقليل وسرّحها على شكل ذيل الفرس. (الصورة ٢) • أربط شريط حول قاعدة ذيل الفرس (الصورة ٣) • إفتل ذيل الفرس بإتجاه جانب الوجه مع لف الشريط في نفس الوقت بالإتجاه المعاكس (الصورة ٤) • أضف خصلة أخرى عن طريق تجميع الشعر من تحت الجديلة وفوقها. كرر ذلك (الصورتين ٥ الى ٦) • تابع ربط الشريط بالإتجاه المعاكس خصلة بعد خصلة (الصورتين ٧ الى ٨) • ثبّت طرف الجديلة الى قاعدة ذيل الفرس (الصورة ٩) • ضع ذيل الجديلة رجوعاً فوق ذروة الرأس لتجلس داخل الدائرة (الصورة ١٠). أربط الشريط على شكل عقدة (الصورة ١١).

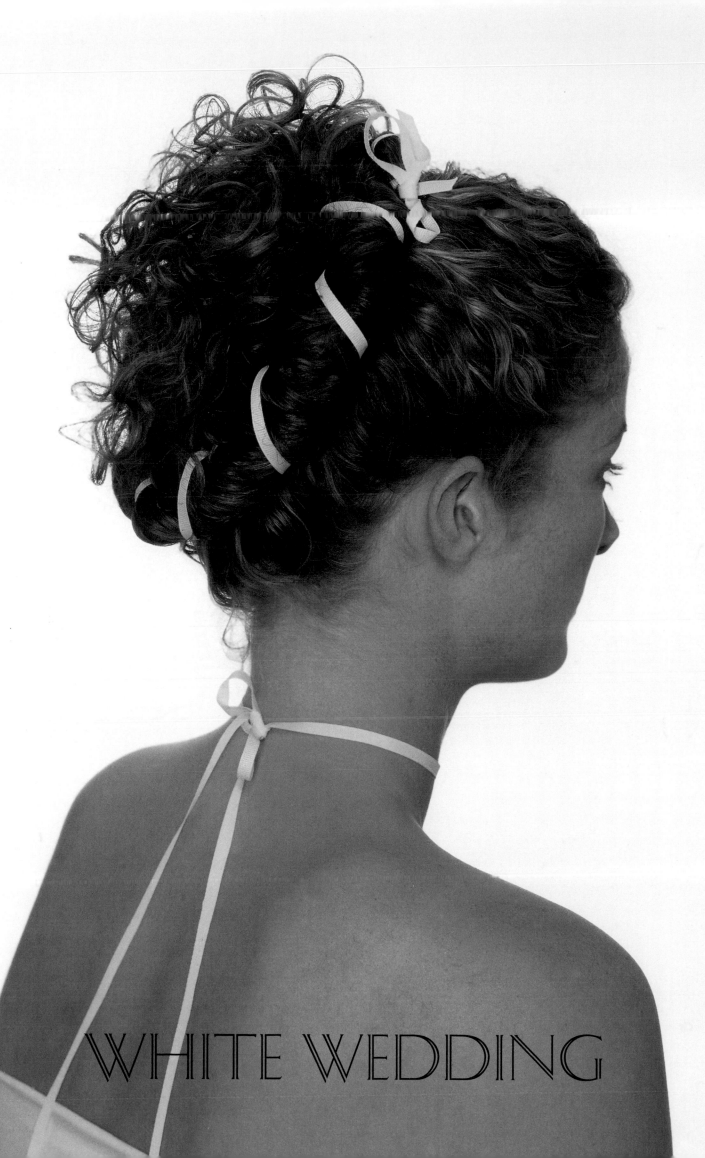

WHITE WEDDING

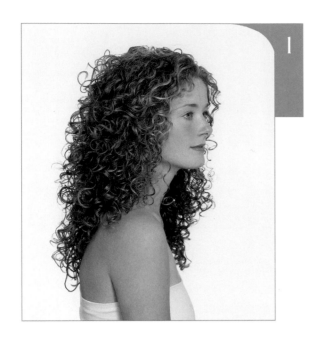

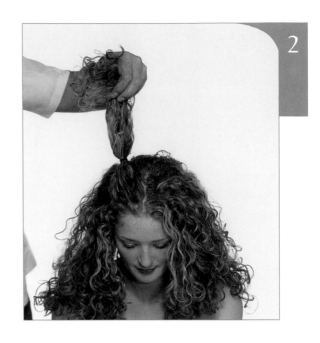

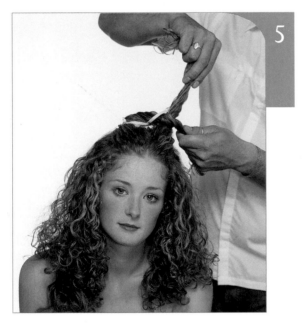

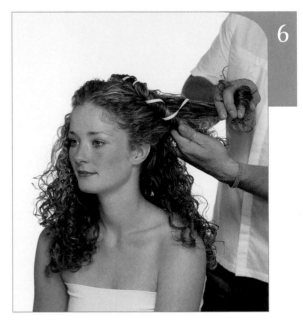

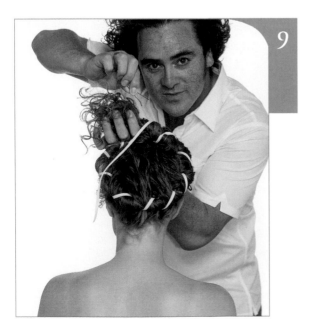

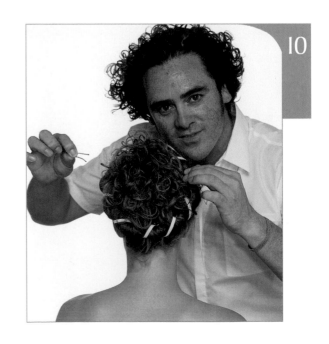

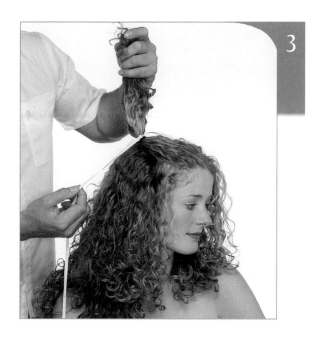

3

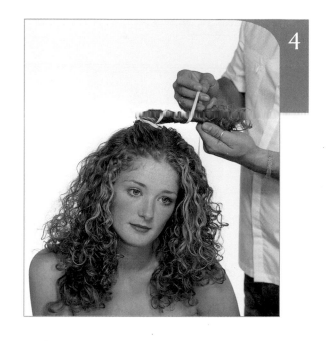

4

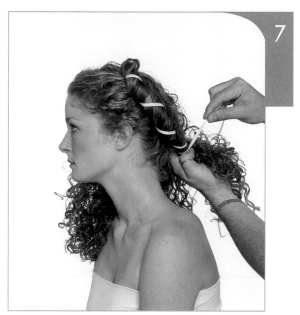

7

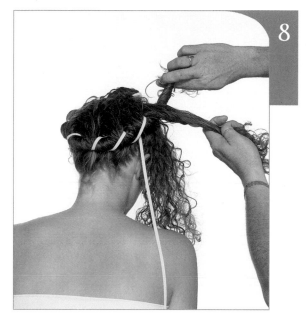

8

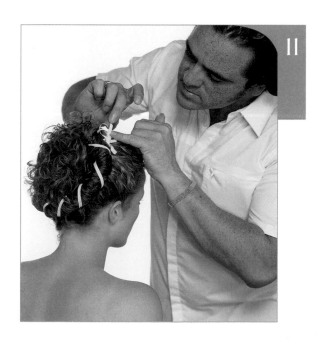

11

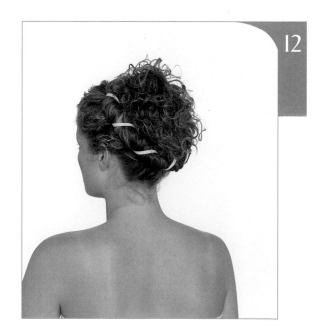

12

WHITE MAGIC

• Take three strands of hair starting 2cm away from front hairline (fig. 2) • Take another strand of hair from the front and place it under using a section clip to hold (fig. 3-4) • Take two more strands from in between then another from the front and again place under. • Repeat all the previous steps to complete a basket weave (fig. 5-9) • Twist all the ends together and pin (fig. 10-11) • Repeat on opposite side (fig. 12-17) • Split back into two and twist both sides into centre. Pin to hold (fig. 18-22) • Backcomb tails and shape, pinning ends into neck (fig. 23-25)

• Drei Haarsträhnen 2 cm von der vorderen Haarlinie entfernt in die Hand nehmen (Abb. 2) • Eine andere Haarsträhne von vorne darunter durchführen und mit einem Clip festheften (Abb. 3-4) • Zwei weitere Strähnen dazwischen und eine weitere von vorne mit einem Clip festheften. • Vorgänge wiederholen, um die Haare fertig zu flechten (Abb. 5-9) • Alle Enden miteinander verdrehen und feststecken (Abb. 10-11) • Vorgang auf der gegenüberliegenden Seite wiederholen (Abb. 12-17) • Haarpartien an der Mittellinie teilen und beide Seiten zur Mitte hin drehen. Feststecken (Abb. 18-22) • Spitzen toupieren und in Form zupfen, Enden am Nacken feststecken (Abb. 23-25)

• Prendere tre ciocche iniziando a 2cm di distanza dall'attaccatura frontale (figura 2) • Prendere un'altra ciocca dalla zona frontale e passarla sotto e fermare (figure 3-4) • Prendere due ciocche dagli spazi intermedi e un'altra dalla zona frontale e portarla indietro e fermare • Ripetere tutti i passaggi precedenti per creare un effetto a intreccio (figure 5-9) • Attorcigliare le ciocche insieme e fermare (figure 10-11) • Ripetere sul lato opposto (figure 12-17) • Dividere in due e attorcigliare entrambii lati al centro e fermare (figure 18-22) • Cotonare le code e disporre le punte verso la nuca e fermare (figure 23-25)

• Prenez trois mèches de cheveux en commençant à 2 cm des racines sur le devant (fig. 2) • Prenez une autre mèche de cheveux sur le devant et placez-la en dessous en la maintenant avec une pince (fig. 3-4) • Prenez deux autres mèches de cheveux dans l'espace intermédiaire et une autre sur le devant et maintenez-les avec une pince. • Répétez la procédure précédente de manière à former un motif en treillis (fig. 5-9) • Enroulez ensemble toutes les extrémités et épinglez (fig. 10-11) • Répétez la procédure de l'autre côté (fig. 12-17) • Divisez en deux et enroulez les deux côtés dans le centre. Maintenir à l'aide d'une épingle (fig. 18-22) • Peignez les queues en arrière et modelez, en fixant les extrémités dans le cou à l'aide d'une épingle. (fig. 23-25)

• Tomar tres mechones de cabello empezando a 2 cm. de distancia de la línea del cabello. (Fig. 2) • Tomar otro mechón de cabello de la parte frontal y colocarla por debajo sujetándola con un clip. (Fig. 3-4) • Tomar otros dos mechones de entre medio y otro de la parte delantera y sujetar con un clip. • Repetir los pasos anteriores hasta completar una trama tejida. (Fig. 5-9) • Enrollar todas las puntas juntas y sujetar con clips. (Fig. 10-11) • Repetir en el lado opuesto. (Fig. 12-17) • Separar la parte posterior en dos y enrollar ambos lados hacia el centro. Sujetar con clips. (Fig. 18-22) • Peinar las colas hacia atrás y dar forma, sujetando con clips las puntas al cuello. (Fig. 23-25)

•フロントの生え際の2cm離れたところから三束とる。（図2）•フロントからもう一束とり、下において、セクションクリップでおさえる。（図3-4）• 間から二束とり、フロントから一束とってセクションクリップでおさえる。•ここまでの全段階を繰り返しバスケット編みを完成させる。（図5-9）。•先端部分をすべてツイストしてピンで留める。（図10-11）•反対側も同様に行う。（図12-17）•バックを二つに分け、両サイドをセンターにツイストする。ピンで固定する。（図18-22）•テールをバックコームして逆毛を立て、形を整える。先端部分はネックに向けてピンで留める。（図23-25）

•离前发线2厘米处取三缕头发(图2) •从前发取另一缕置于下面，用发夹固定(图3-4) •之间再取两缕，又从前发取一缕，发夹固定 •重复前面步骤以形成一个篮子编织图案(图5-9) •编结所有底发，夹住(图10-11) •另一边重复(图12-17) •后发分成两部份，向中央编结。发夹固定(图18-22) •逆梳发梢造型，尾端夹入颈部(图23-25)

• إلتقط ثلاث ضفائر من الشعر إبتداء من مسافة ٢ سم وراء حد الشعر الأمامي (الصورة ٢) • خذ ضفيرة أخرى من الأمام وشدها تحت الضفائر الجانبية مع تثبيتها بواسطة ملقط (الصورتين ٣ و٤) • إلتقط ضفيرتين أخريين من المسا حة الوسطى للشعر وضفيرة أخرى من الأمام وثبتها معاً بواسطة ملقط. • كرر جميع الخطوات المذكورة أعلاه لحياكة الشعر على شكل سلة (الصور ٥ الى ٩) • إفتل جميع الأطراف سوياً وثبتها بدبابيس (الصورتين ١٠ و١١) • كرر نفس الإجراء على الجانب الآخر (الصور ١٢ الى ١٧) • إقسم الجزء الخلفي من الشعر الى قسمين وإفتل القسمين باتجاه منتصف الرأس. ثبت بدبابيس (الصورتين ١٨ الى ٢٢) • مشّط الذيول بالإتجاه المعاكس وشكّلها مع تثبيت الأطراف على الرقبة بواسطة دبابيس (الصور ٢٣ الى ٢٥)

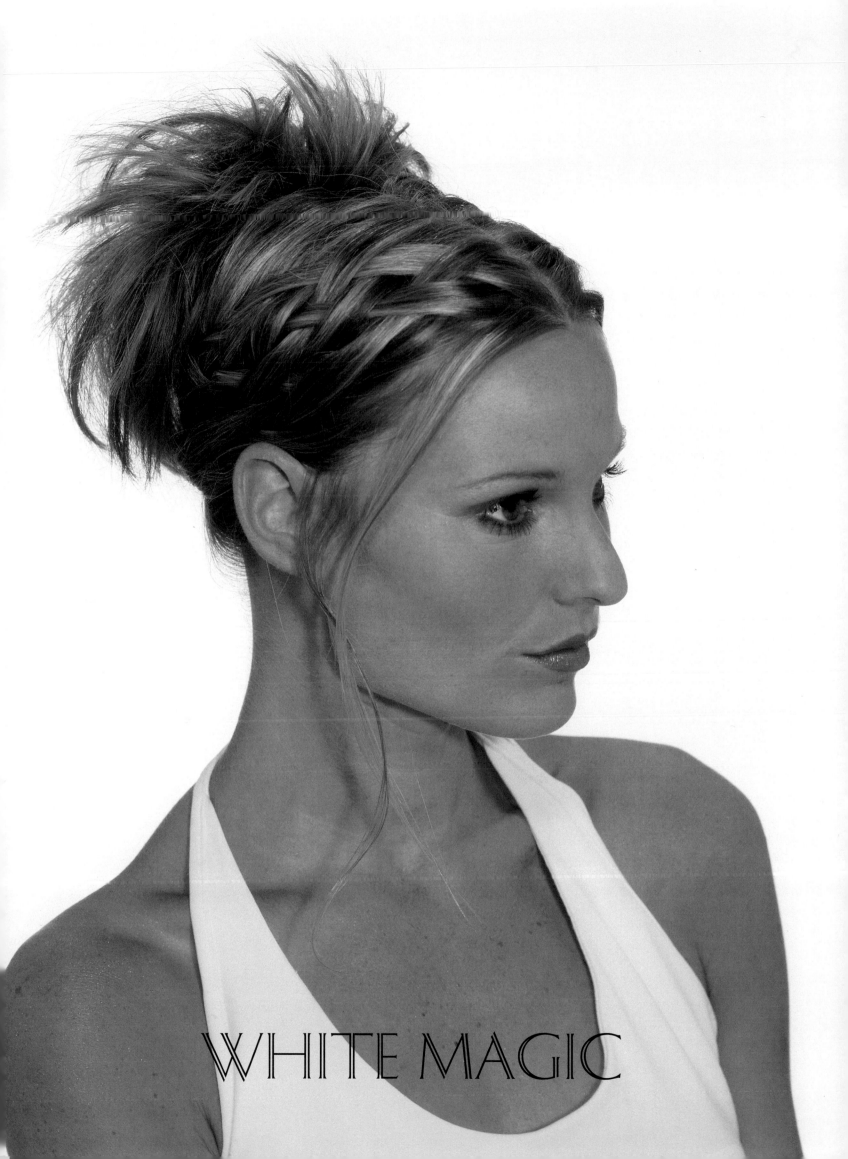

WHITE MAGIC

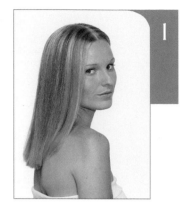

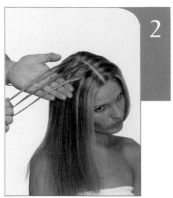

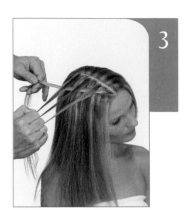

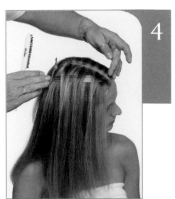

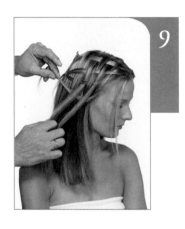

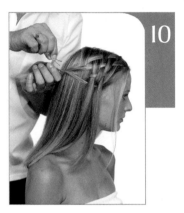

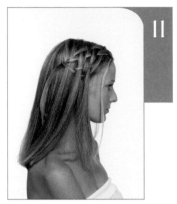

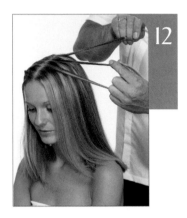

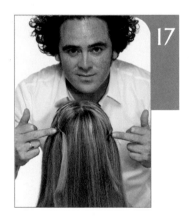

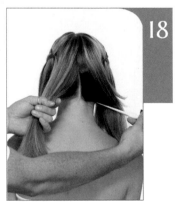

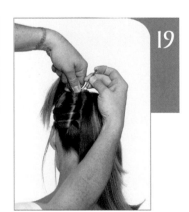

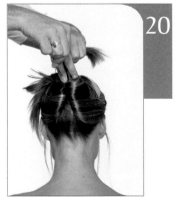

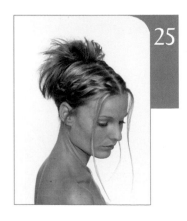

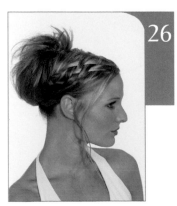

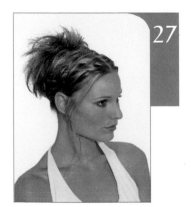

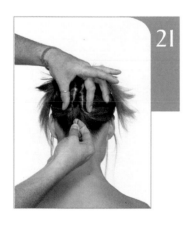

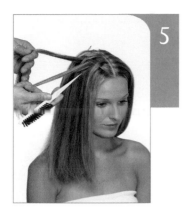

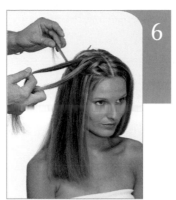

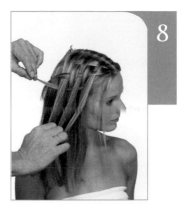

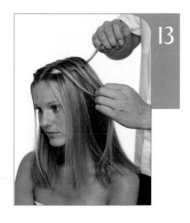

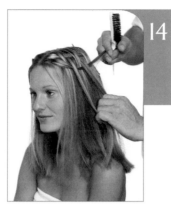

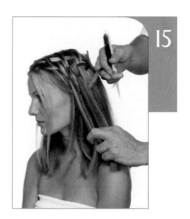

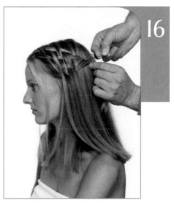

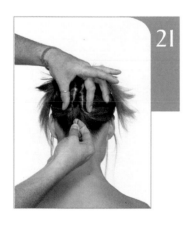

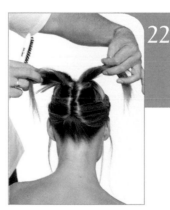

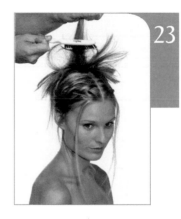

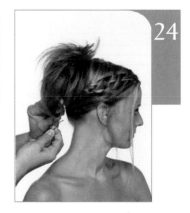

WHITE ICE

• Section front and back and place back into ponytail below crown (fig. 2) •Place hair band halfway down ponytail (fig. 3) • Backcomb tail and roll forward with backcombed area inside. Pin in front of ponytail base (fig. 4-7) • Set front area with hot rollers (fig. 8-10) • Brush front areas (except fringe) back and plait. Lift plait over base and pin to hold (fig. 11-14) • Place tails over base for softness (fig. 15) • Drape fringe area over base and spray (fig. 16-17)

• Haare in zwei seitliche Zöpfe und einen Pferdeschwanz unter dem Scheitel abtrennen (Abb. 2) • Haargummi auf halber Länge des Pferdeschwanzes anbringen (Abb. 3) • Pferdeschwanz toupieren und nach vorne rollen, so dass der toupierte Haarabschnitt innen ist. Vor dem Ansatz des Pferdeschwanzes feststecken (Abb. 4-7) • Die beiden seitlichen Zöpfe auf heißen Lockenwicklern aufwickeln (Abb. 8-10) • Die seitlichen Haare (ausgenommen des Ponys) zurückkämmen und flechten. Nun den geflochtenen Zopf über das Unterhaar legen und feststecken (Abb. 11-14) • Verschiedene Strähnen über das Unterhaar legen, um dem Ganzen etwas mehr Weichheit zu verleihen (Abb. 15) • Nun die Ponyhaare über dem Unterhaar drapieren und mit Haarspray festsprühen (Abb. 16-17)

• Separare la parte anteriore e quella posteriore mettendo quest'ultima in una coda sulla sommita' del capo (figura 2) • Mettere un elastico a meta' coda (figura 3) • Cotonare la coda e arrotolarla in avanti con la parte cotonata all'interno. Fermare sul davanti nella base della coda (figure 4-7) • Mettere dei bigodini caldi sulla parte anteriore (figura 8-10) • Spazzolare la zona frontale (eccetto la frangia) all'indietro e intrecciare. Disporre la treccia sopra la base e fermare (figure 11-14) • Mettere le punte sopra la base per dare morbidezza (figura 15) • Riportare la frangia sulla base e spruzzare (figure 16-17)

• Séparez l'avant et l'arrière et mettez l'arrière en queue de cheval sous le haut de la tête (fig. 2) • Placez le bandeau sur le milieu de la queue de cheval (fig. 3) • Peignez la queue en arrière et roulez sur le devant avec la section peignée vers l'intérieur. Epinglez sur le devant de la base de la queue de cheval (fig. 4-7) • Traitez la section avant avec des rouleaux chauds (fig. 8-10) • Brossez la section avant (sauf la frange) vers l'arrière et nattez. Placez la natte sur la base et maintenez à l'aide d'une épingle (fig. 11-14) • Placez les queues sur la base pour la douceur (fig. 15) • Drapez la frange sur la base et vaporisez (fig. 16-17)

• Separar la parte delantera de la parte trasera y hacer una cola con la parte posterior por debajo de la coronilla. (Fig. 2) • Colocar una goma para el cabello a la mitad de la cola. (Fig. 3) • Peinar la cola hacia atrás y enrollar hacia delante con la zona peinada en la parte interior. Sujetar con clips la parte frontal de la base de la cola. (Fig. 4-7) • Aplicar rulos calientes en la parte delantera. (Fig. 8-10) • Cepillar la parte delantera (excepto el flequillo) hacia atrás y trenzar. Levantar la trenza sobre la pase y sujetar con un clip. (Fig. 11-14) • Colocar trenzas sobre la base para añadir suavidad. (Fig. 15) • Dejar caer el flequillo sobre la base y aplicar laca. (Fig. 16-17)

• フロントとバックに分け、バックはクラウンの下でポニーテールを作る。(図2) • ポニーテールの途中真ん中をヘアバンドで結ぶ。(図3)
• テールをバックコームで逆毛を立て、逆毛にした箇所を内側にしながら前方へ巻く。ポニーテール・ベースの前にピンで留める。(図4-7)
• ホットローラーでフロントをセットする。(図8-10) • フロント(フリンジは除く)をバックへブラッシングして、みつ編みにする。編み下げをベースの上へ持ち上げ、ピンで固定する。(図11-14) • テールをベースの上に持ってきて、やわらかい感じをだす。(図15) • ベースの上にフリンジをたらし、スプレーをかける。(図16-17)

• 分开前后头发，在头顶下方，将后面头发扎成马尾(图2) • 在马尾半中扎发带(图3) • 逆梳马尾，向前翻卷，逆梳的部份在内，夹在马尾发根的前面(图4-7)
• 前面的头发夹上热卷发筒(图8-10) • 逆梳梳前面头发部份(流苏除外)，结成辫。将辫举向发基，夹住(图11-14) • 将马尾移到发基(图15) • 将流苏披向发基，喷发胶(图16-17)

• إقسم الشعر الى قسمين أمامي وخلفي، إجمع القسم الخلفي على شكل ذيل الفرس (الصورة ٢) • ضع ربطة الشعر في منتصف ذيل الفرس (الصورة ٣)
• مشّط ذيل الفرس بالإتجاه المعاكس ثم لفّه نحو الأمام بحيث يكون الشعر الذي مشطّه هكذا على الجانب الداخلي من اللفة. ثبته بالدبابيس أمام قاعدة ذيل الفرس (الصور ٤ الى ٧) • صفف القسم الأمامي على لفات مسخنة كهربائياً (الصور ٨ الى ١٠) • مشّط القسم الأمامي (ما عدا الأطراف) نحو الخلف ثم أجدله. إرفع الجديلة فوق قاعدة ذيل الفرس وثبتها بدبابيس (الصور ١١ الى ١٤) • ضع الذيول فوق القاعدة لإضافة مظهر ناعم (الصورة ١٥) • إرخي أطراف الشعر الأمامية فوق التسريحة ثم رشها (الصورتين ١٦ و١٧)

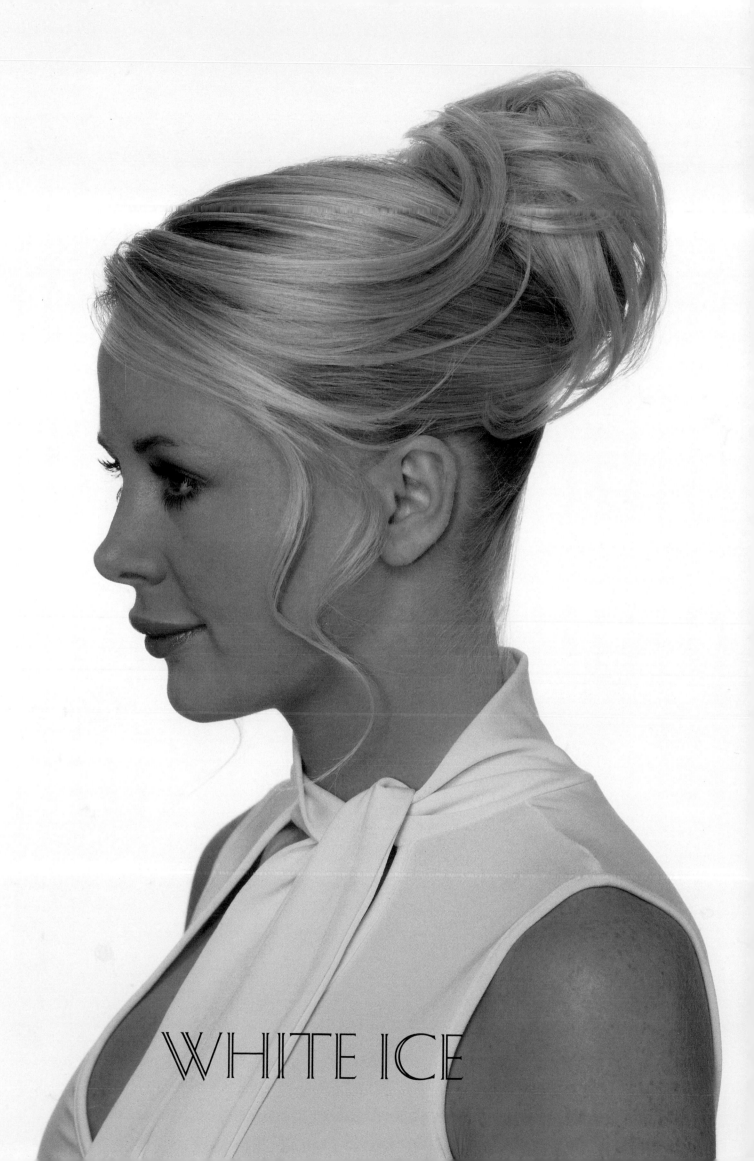

WHITE ICE

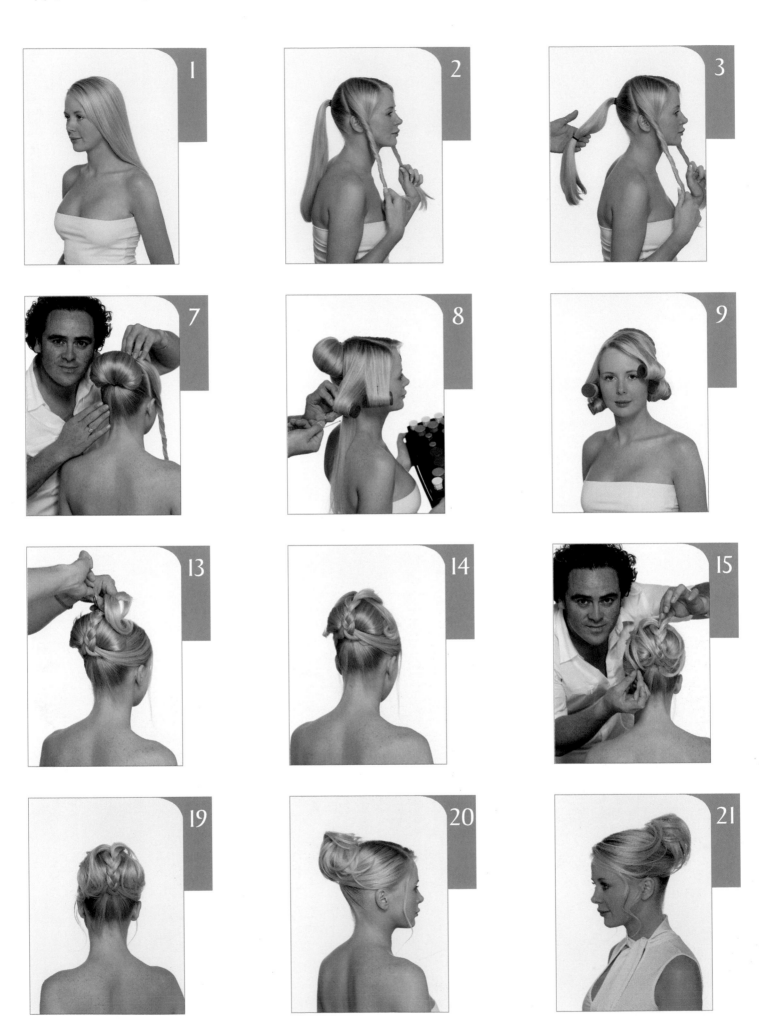

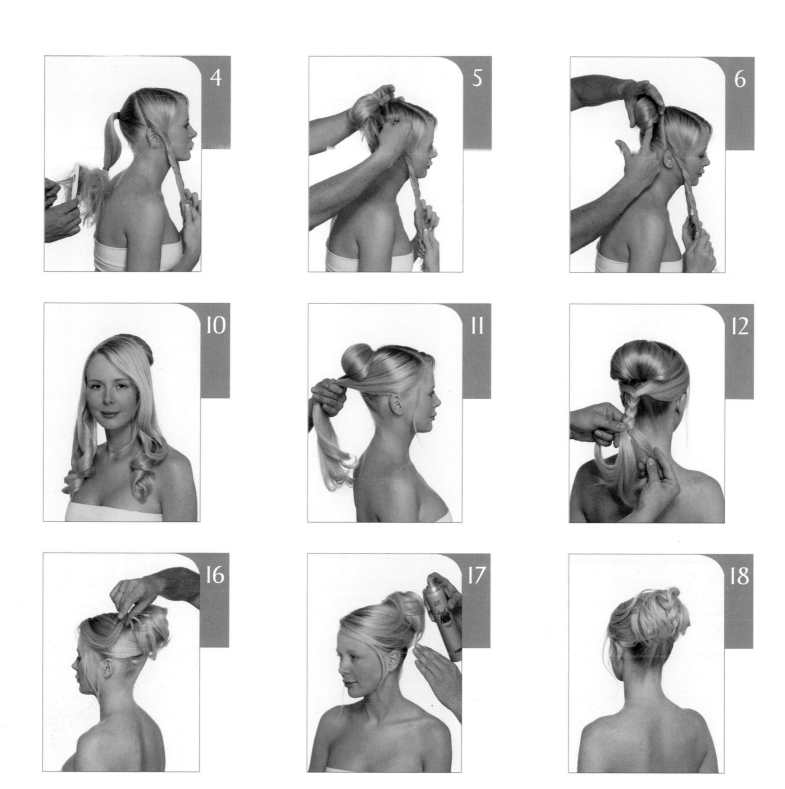

WHITE CLOUD

• Colour tone hair weft to match client's hair colour (see page 73) (fig. 1) • Section area around head, below crown (fig. 2) • Scalp braid from side to side. Fold braid back to middle and pin (fig. 3-5) • Pin base of hairpiece to braid, across to other side and back again (fig. 6-8) • Place top hair over hair weft and spray (fig. 9) • Take side section and treat with product (fig. 10) • Twist and pin side section behind ear on both sides (fig. 11-12) • Take another slice with pinned section and twist (fig. 13-14) • Take a small thread of hair and hold while pushing twist back toward scalp. Pin. (fig. 15-17) • Repeat all the way around the head (fig. 18-26) • Take front area and drape back (fig. 27)

• Farblich passendes Haarstück einsetzen (siehe Seite 73) (Abb. 1) • Haarabschnitt um den Kopf herum unter dem Scheitel einteilen (Abb. 2) • Von einer Seite zur anderen flechten. Flechtschwanz zurück zur Mitte legen und feststecken (Abb. 3-5) • Den Ansatz des Haarstückes am Flechtschwanz feststecken, hinüber zur anderen Seite und wieder zurück (Abb. 6-8) • Oberhaar mit einer Haarklammer festhalten und mit Haarspray festsprühen (Abb. 9) • Auf eine Haarsträhne Gel/Mousse geben (Abb. 10) • Drehen und seitlichen Haarabschnitt auf beiden Seiten hinter den Ohren feststecken (Abb. 11-12) • Einen weiteren Haarabschnitt drehen (Abb. 13-14) • Eine kleine Haarsträhne festhalten, dabei die verdrehte Strähne zurück zur Kopfhaut schieben. Feststecken. (Abb. 15-17) • Den gleichen Vorgang rund um den Kopf herum wiederholen (Abb. 18-26) • Nun die vorderen Haare nach hinten drapieren (Abb. 27)

• Colorare il posticcio (vedi pagina 73) del colore della cliente (figura 1) • Separare una zona sotto la sommita' del capo (figura 2) • Eseguire una treccia attaccata piegando poi la treccia all'interno e fermare (figure 3-5) • Assicurare il posticcio sulla lunghezza della treccia base (figure 6-8) • Disporre i capelli della sommita' sopra la base del posticcio e spruzzare (figura 9) • Prendere i capelli della zona laterale e applicare il prodotto (figura 10) • Attorcigliare e fermare dietro l'orecchio su entrambi i lati (figure 11-12) • Prender una ciocca e attorcigliare (figure 13-14) • Separare una piccolissima quantita' di capelli tenendoli mentre spingete i capelli attorcigliati verso la cute, e fermare. (figure 15-17) • Ripetere questo passaggio intorno alla testa (figure 18-26) • Riportare la zona frontale all'indietro (figura 27)

• Colorez une mèche de cheveux (voir page 73) (fig. 1) • Séparez une section sur le pourtour de la tête, sous le haut de la tête (fig. 2) • Nattez jusqu'au cuir chevelu d'un côté sur l'autre. Repliez la natte sur le milieu et épinglez (fig. 3-5) • Epinglez la base de la mèche postiche sur la natte, en croisant puis en revenant du premier côté (fig. 6-8) • Placez les cheveux du dessus sur la mèche de cheveux et vaporisez (fig. 9) • Prenez la section latérale et traitez au produit (fig. 10) • Enroulez et épinglez la section latérale derrière l'oreille des deux côtés (fig. 11-12) • Prenez une autre section et enroulez (fig. 13-14) • Prenez une petite mèche de cheveux et tenez-la tout en poussant et en réenroulant vers le cuir chevelu. Epinglez. (fig. 15-17) • Répétez la procédure tout autour de la tête (fig. 18-26) • Prenez la section avant et drapez-la sur l'arrière (fig. 27)

• Teñir el postizo para que el color sea el mismo que el del cabello de la clienta (ver página 73). (Fig. 1) • Separar una sección de cabello alrededor de la cabeza, por debajo de la coronilla. (Fig. 2) • Trenzar de lado a lado. Doblar la trenza a la mitad y sujetar con un clip. (Fig. 3-5) • Sujetar con clips la base del cabello hasta la trenza, cruzando hacia el otro lado y volviendo al principio. (Fig. 6-8) • Colocar la parte superior del cabello sobre el postizo y rociar con laca. (Fig. 9) • Tomar la sección lateral y aplicar producto. (Fig. 10) • Enrollar y sujetar con un clip la sección de detrás de la oreja a ambos lados. (Fig. 11-12) • Tomar otra sección y enrollar. (Fig. 13-14) • Tomar un pequeño mechón de cabello y sujetar mientras se enrolla hacia atrás. Sujetar con un clip. (Fig. 15-17) • Repetir en toda la cabeza. (Fig. 18-26) • Tomar al parte frontal y dejar caer hacia atrás. (Fig. 27)

• クライアントのヘアカラーに合わせて、ヘアピースにカラーを入れる。（73ページを参照のこ）(図1) • クラウンの下でヘッド全体を分ける。(図2) • 頭皮にそってサイドからサイドにかけて編む。編んだ髪を中央へ折り返し、ピンで留める(図3-5) • ヘアピースのベースを編んだ髪にピンで留め、反対側へ渡した後、戻す。(図6-8) • トップヘアをヘアピースの上に持ってきてスプレーをかける。(図9) • サイドセクションをとり、トリートメント剤で整える。(図10) • サイドセクションをツイストして両側の耳の後ろにピンで留める。(図11-12) • 次にまた一すじとり、ツイストする。(図13-14) • 細い一すじのヘアをとり、ツイストを頭皮に向かって押しながら固定する。ピンで留める。(図15-17) • ヘッド全体を同様に行う。(図18-26) • フロントヘアを後ろへ流す。(図27)

• 给发纬上色(见页73)(图1) • 在头顶下面，取一片头发(图2) • 一边一边地结辫. 将辫折向中间，夹住(图3-5) • 将基发夹向辫子，穿到另一边，再折回(图6-8) • 将头顶头发带到发纬，喷发胶(图9) • 旁边头发用发剂处理(图10) • 两边耳朵后的头发编结，夹住(图11-12) • 取一缕头发，编结(图13-14) • 取一小缕头发，拿住，同时将编结向后推，夹住(图15-17) • 重复头顶周围(图18-26) • 将头顶的头发向后披(图27)

• إختر الشعر المستعار بلون يناسب الشعر الذي يجري تسريحه (أنظر صفحة ٧٣) (الصورة ١) • إقسم الشعر الى خصل إبتداء من ذروة الرأس (الصورة ٢) • إجدل الشعر بشدة من الجانبين لتكوين جديلة متحاذية مع فروة الرأس ثم إطويها نحو الخلف الى وسط الرأس وثبتها بدبابيس (الصور ٣ الى ٥) • اربط قاعدة الشعر المستعار الى الجديلة من جهة الى أخرى (الصور ٦ الى ٨) • ضع الشعر العلوي فوق الشعر المستعار ورشه (الصورة ٩) • خذ خصلة جانبية وضع منتج التصفيف عليها (الصورة ١٠) • إفتل الخصلة الجانبية وثبتها وراء الأذن على جهتي الرأس (الصورتين ١١ و١٢) • خذ خصلة أخرى وإفتلها (الصورتين ١٣ و١٤) • إمسك خيط رفيع من الشعر بينما تدفع بالخصلة الملفوفة نحو فروة الرأس. ثبتها بدبابيس (الصور ١٥ الى ١٧) • كرر هذه العملية على كل الشعر الباقي حول الرأس (الصور ١٨ الى ٢٦) • أسدل الآن الشعر الأمامي نحو الخلف (الصورة ٢٧)

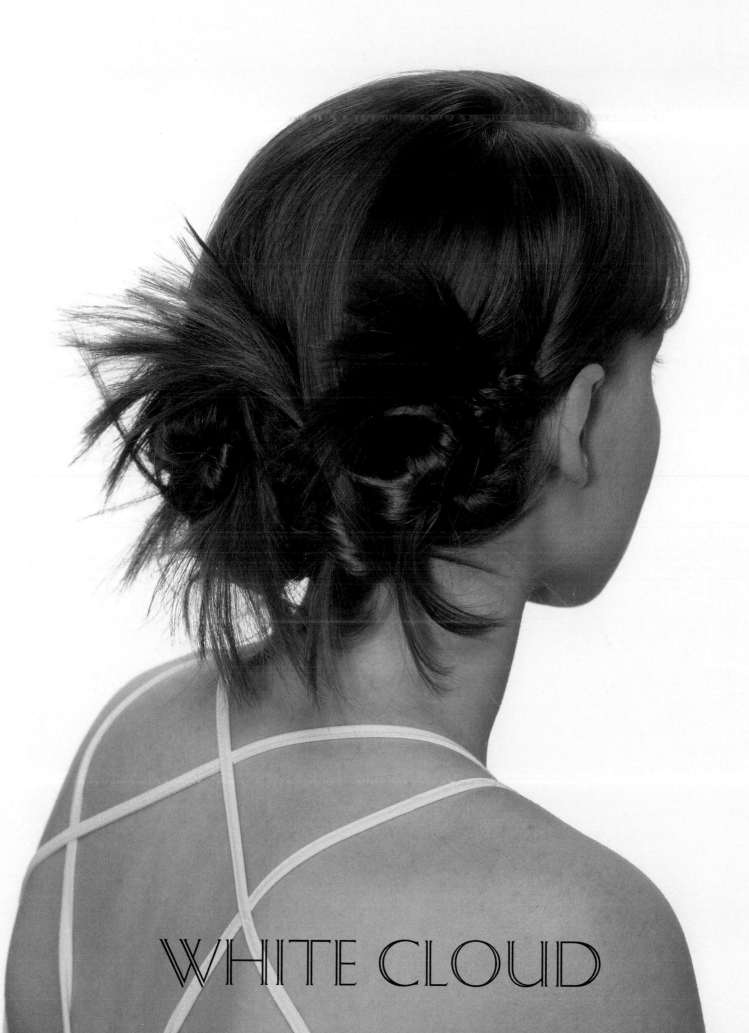

WHITE CLOUD

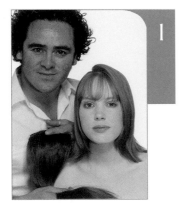

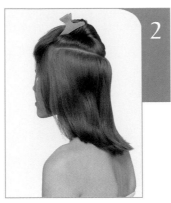

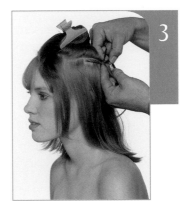

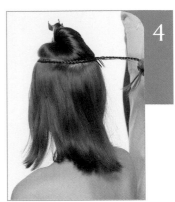

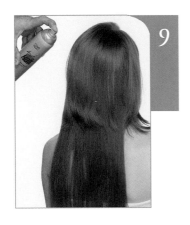

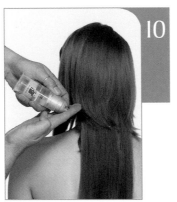

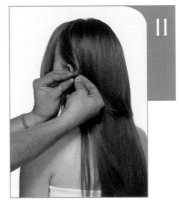

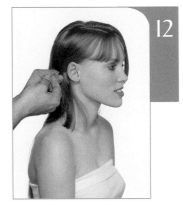

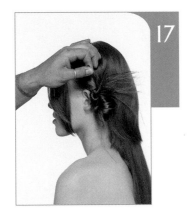

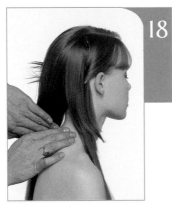

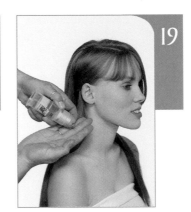

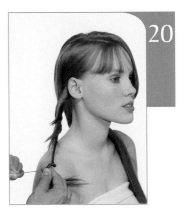

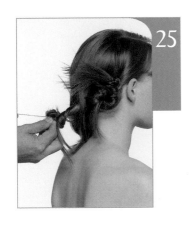

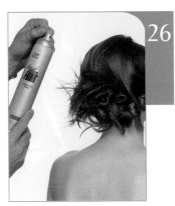

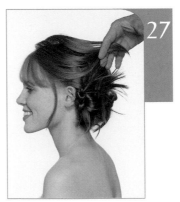

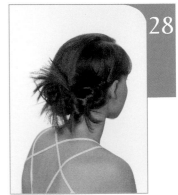

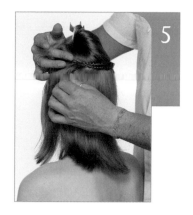

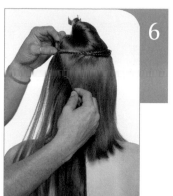

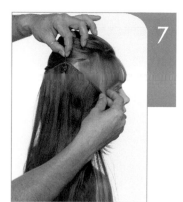

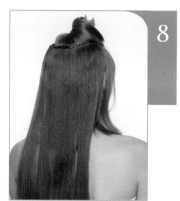

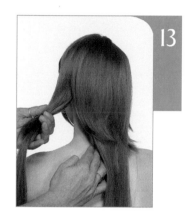

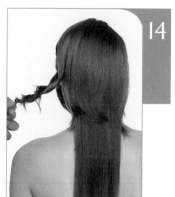

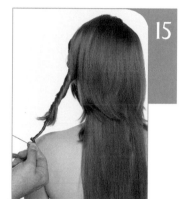

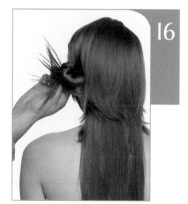

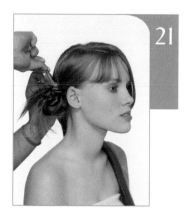

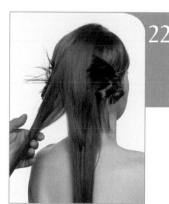

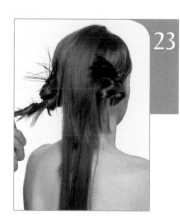

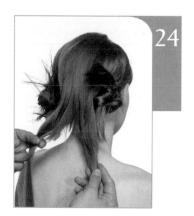

WHITE SNOW

• Section hair from ear to crown to ear and place into ponytail at nape of neck (fig. 3) • Place hair band halfway down ponytail (fig. 4) • Backcomb tail and roll forward with backcombed area inside. Pin above of ponytail base and create crescent shape (fig. 5-9) • Brush front section back over crown, twist down to nape of neck and pin (fig. 10-13) • Split tail into two, backcomb and smooth with brush (fig. 14-16) • Tuck and wrap under base and pin up into nape. Repeat on opposite side.(fig. 17-19) • Spray and blow-dry simultaneously (high heat, slow speed) to set for extra hold (fig. 20)

• Die Haare von den Ohren und dem Scheitel kämmen und im Nacken zum Pferdeschwanz zusammenbinden (Abb. 3) • Etwa auf halber Länge des Pferdeschwanzes das Haarband befestigen (Abb. 4) • Das Schwanzende toupieren und nach vorne einrollen, so dass die toupierten Haare innen liegen. Die Haare über dem Ansatz des Pferdeschwanzes halbmondförmig feststecken (Abb. 5-9) • Nun die Seitenhaare über den Scheitel nach hinten kämmen, bis zum Nacken verzwirbeln und feststecken (Abb. 10-13) • Den Pferdeschwanz in zwei Strähnen unterteilen, toupieren und glatt bürsten (Abb. 14-16) • Haare unter dem Ansatz und dann im Nacken feststecken. Den Vorgang auf der gegenüberliegenden Seite wiederholen (Abb. 17-19) • Haare langsam aber bei hoher Hitze föhnen und gleichzeitig mit Haarspray fixieren, um so für zusätzlichen Halt zu sorgen (Abb. 20)

• Separare i capelli da orecchio, sommita', orecchio e fare una coda sulla nuca (figura 3) • Mettere un elastico a meta' coda (figura 4) • Cotonare la coda e avvolgere in avanti con la parte cotonata all'interno, fermare sulla base della coda creando una mezza luna (figure 5-9) • Spazzolare la zona frontale all'indietro, attorcigliare verso il basso e fermare (figure 10-13) • Dividere la coda in due, cotonare e spazzolare leggermente (figure 14-16) • Avvolgere e inserire le punte sotto la base e fermare sulla nuca. Ripetendo il passaggio con il lato opposto (figure 17-19) • Spruzzare utilizzando il phon contemporaneamente (calore massimo ,velocita' minima) per una tenuta piu' forte (figura 20)

• Séparez les cheveux de l'oreille au haut de la tête et à l'oreille et faites une queue de cheval sur la nuque (fig. 3) • Placez un bandeau à mi-hauteur sur la queue de cheval (fig. 4) • Peignez vers l'arrière et roulez vers l'avant avec la partie peignée à l'intérieur. Epinglez au-dessus de la base de la queue de cheval et arrangez les cheveux en forme de croissant (fig. 5-9) • Brossez la section de devant vers l'arrière par-dessus le haut de la tête, enroulez sur la nuque et épinglez (fig. 10-13) • Séparez la queue de cheval en deux, peignez vers l'arrière et finissez à la brosse (fig. 14-16) • Serrez et enroulez sous la base et épinglez sur la nuque. Répétez la procédure du côté opposé (fig. 17-19) • Vaporisez et séchez simultanément (très chaud, faible vitesse) pour assurer un bon maintien (fig. 20).

• Separar una sección del cabello desde la oreja hasta la coronilla y atar en una cola en la base del cuello. (Fig. 3) • Colocar una goma para el pelo a la mitad de la cola. (Fig. 4) • Peinar la cola al revés y enrollar hacia delante de forma que la zona peinada quede en el interior. Sujetar con clips por encima de la base de la cola y crear una forma de media luna. (Fig. 5-9) • Cepillar la sección frontal hacia atrás sobre la coronilla, retorcer enrollando el cabello hasta la base del cuello y sujetar con clips. (Fig. 10-13) • Dividir la cola en dos partes, peinar al revés y alisar con un cepillo. (Fig. 14-16) • Envolver bajo la base escondiendo las puntas y sujetar con un clip en la parte de la nuca. (Fig. 17-19) • Aplicar laca mientras se seca con el secador de mano (a gran temperatura y poca velocidad) para que quede fijo y sujeto. (Fig. 20)

バックを両耳からクラウンにかけてセクション分けし、えりあしの上でポニーテールを作る。（図３）●ポニーテールの途中真ん中をヘアバンドで結ぶ。（図４）●テールをテールをバックコームで逆毛を立て、逆毛にした箇所を内側にしながら前方へ巻く。ポニーテール・ベースの上で三日月の形にピンで留める。（図５－９）●フロントをクラウンの後ろへブラッシングし、下へツイストしてえりあしでピンで留める。（図10－13））●テールを二つに分け、バックコームで逆毛を立て、ブラシでならす。（図14－16）● ベースの下で巻き付けてしまいこみ、えりあしへピンで留める。反対側も同様に繰り返す。（図17－19）● スプレーをかけながら高温でゆっくりとブローししっかりとホールドするようセットする。（図20）

•将头发从耳鬓到额头再到耳鬓分开，在颈背处拢成发辫（图3）•在发辫中央扎上皮筋（图4）•从前向后梳理发辫，再向前卷起来，梳过的部分卷在里面。在发辫根上方用发夹夹住，形成新月形（图5－9）•将前额部分的头发向后梳，弯到颈背处，用发夹夹住（图10－13）•将发辫分为两缕，用梳子从前向后梳理，令其平整（图14－16）•卷起来，包在发髻底端，用发夹固定。另一侧同样处理（图17－19）•喷上发胶，同时吹干（热风，慢速），使其定型（图20）

•قسّن الشعر من الأُذن الى ذروة الرأس والى الأذن ثم جسّده في شكل ذيل الفرس في قفا العنق (الشكل ٣) ● ضع طوق الشعر في نصف طول ذيل الفرس (الشكل ٤)
● امشط الشعر الى الخلف ولفه الى الأمام مع وضع الجزء الخلفي الممشوط في داخل اللفافة. اشبك بالدبوس في قاعدة ذيل الفرس لتكوين شكل هلال (الشكل ٥-٩
● امسح الجزء الأمامى بالفرشاة الى الخلف فوق ذروة الرأس، افتله الى الأسفل على قفا العنق ثم اشبكه بالدبوس (الشكل ١٠-١٣) ● افصل الذيل الى قسمين، امشط
القسم الأول الى الخلف ثم نعّمه بالفرشاة (الشكل ١٤-١٦) ● قم بزم الشعر ولفه تحت القاعدة ثم اشبكه بالدبوس في قفا العنق. كرر ذلك في القسم المواجه
(الشكل ١٧-١٩) ● قم ببخ الشعر وتجفيفه بالهواء الساخن في نفس الوقت (استخدم درجة الحرارة العالية ولكن بسرعة خفيفة) للحصول على تماسك أقوى للشعر
(الشكل ٢٠)

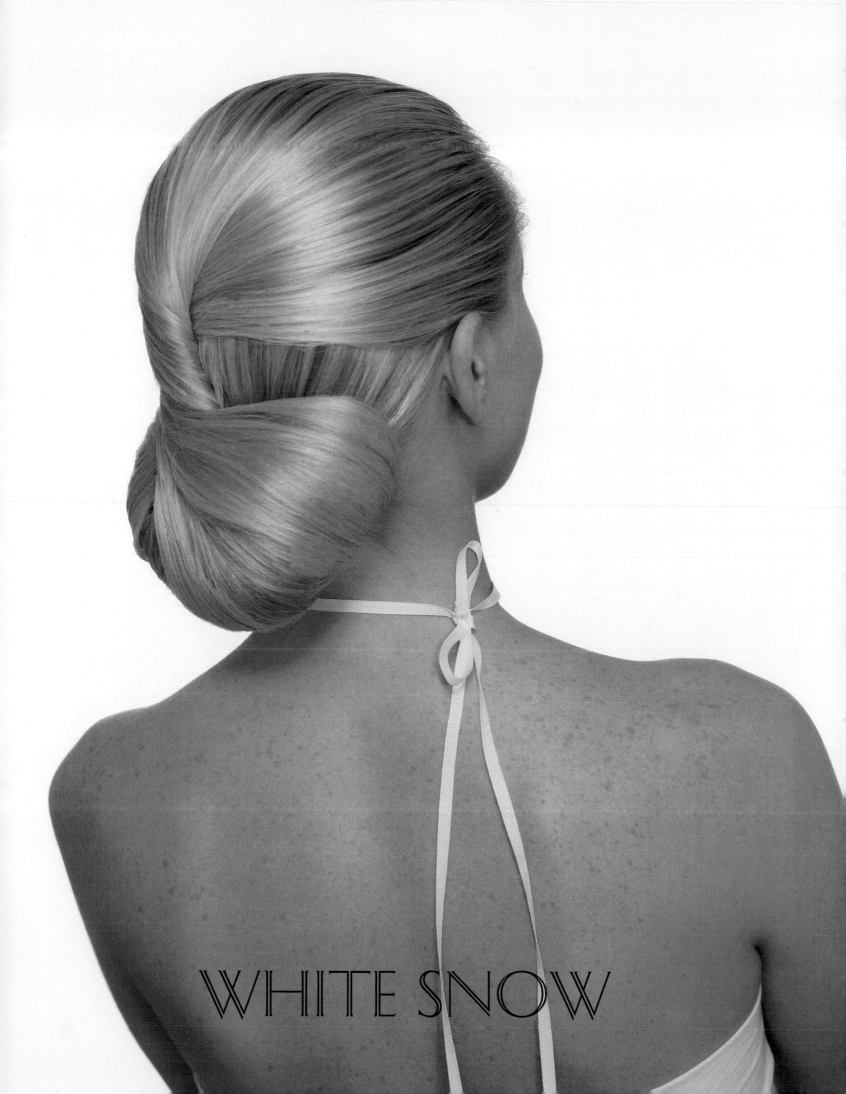

WHITE SNOW

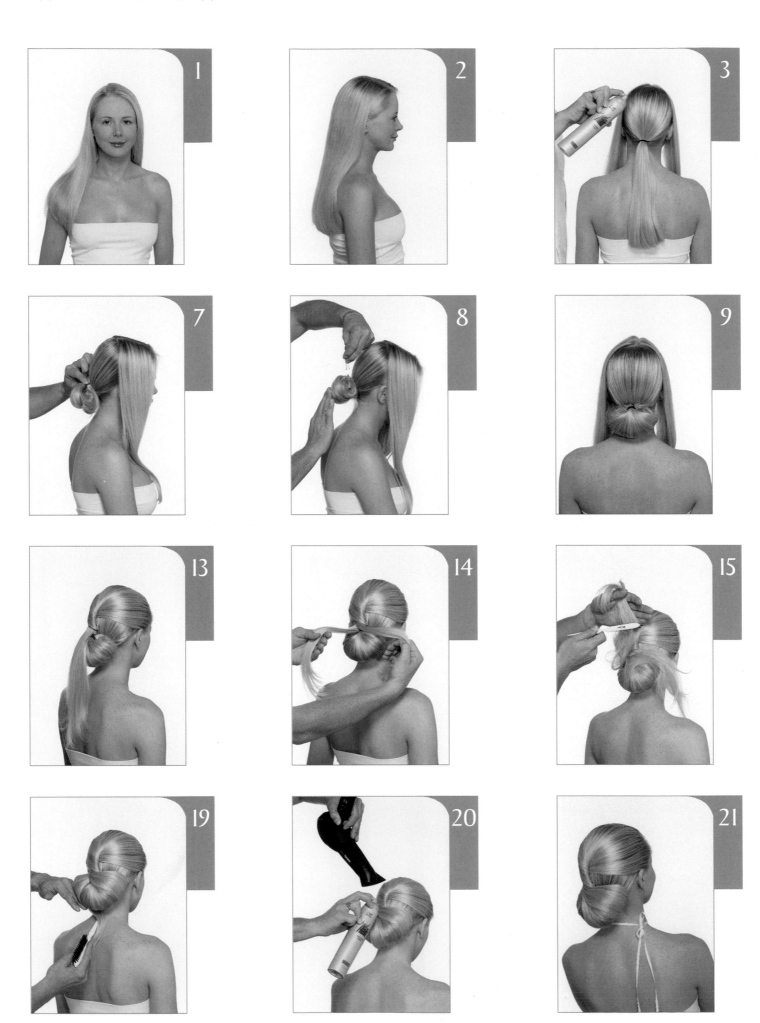

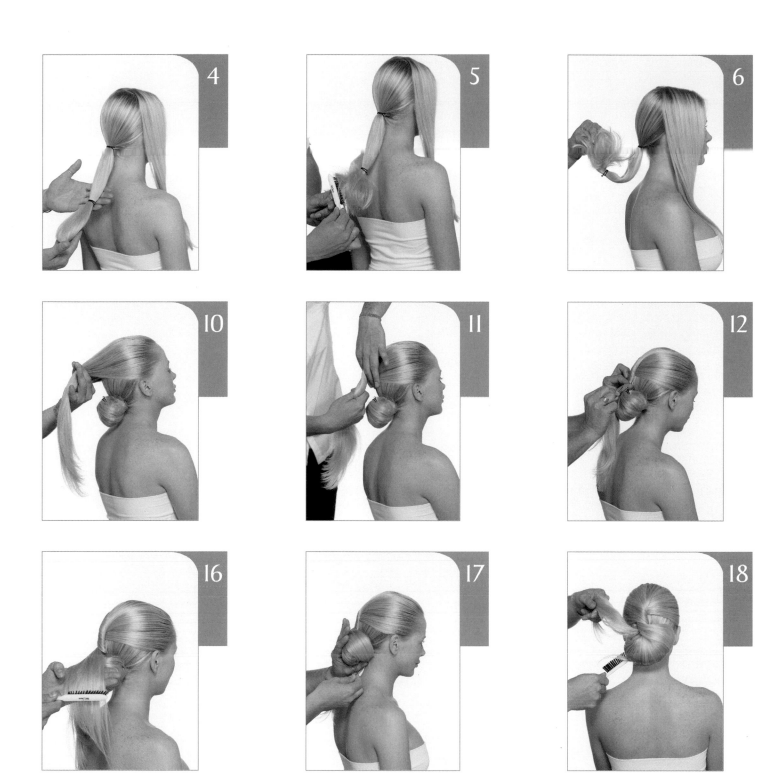

WHITE LILLIES

• Create a triangular section 6cm across crown and down to sharp point at occipital (fig. 2) • Twist tightly to create base and pin, leaving tail out (fig.2-3) • Section top area and get client to hold (fig. 4) • Slice side section and brush to opposite side of base and pin into base. Repeat on other side (fig. 5-8) • Repeat over and over creating a criss-cross pattern (fig. 9-11) • Continue behind ear always taking 45 degree angled sections (fig. 12-16) • Take tails and create loose swirls and pin (fig. 17-18) • Spray to hold (fig.19) • Split top area into two, tie in a knot, let tails swirl on top and pin (fig. 20-24)

• Ein dreieckiges Haarstück 6 cm über dem Scheitel abtrennen, wobei die spitzeste Spitze nach unten geneigt sein sollte (Abb. 2) • Fest verzwirbeln und feststecken, dabei jedoch die Strähne auslassen (Abb.2-3) • Oberhaar abtrennen und die Kundin bitten, es festzuhalten (Abb. 4) • Seitenhaare abtrennen und auf die gegenüberliegende Seite des Unterhaares bürsten und feststecken. Vorgang auf der anderen Seite wiederholen (Abb. 5-8) • Vorgang wiederholen und dabei ein Kreuzlinienmuster schaffen (Abb. 9-11) • Vorgang hinter dem Ohr fortführen und dabei stets 45° geneigte Haarabschnitte verwenden (Abb. 12-16) • Mit den Spitzen lockere Spiralen kreieren und feststecken (Abb. 17-18) • Mit Haarspray in Form sprühen (Abb.19) • Das Oberhaar zweiteilen, verknoten, die Spitzen oben kreiseln lassen und feststecken (Abb. 20-24)

• Creare una sezione triangolare larga circa 6cm sulla sommita'del capo (figura 2) • Attorcigliare strettamente per creare una base e fermare lasciando le punte fuori (figure 2-3) • Separare la parte anteriore e chiedere alla cliente di tenerla (figura 4) • Prendere una ciocca dalla zona laterale e portarla spazzolandola sul lato opposto della base fermandola, ripetere dal lato opposto (figure 5-8) • Ripetere piu' volte creando un motivo a incrocio (figure 9-11) • Continuare dietro l'orecchio con sezioni diagonali a 45 gradi (figure 12-16) • Prendere le punte e formare dei riccioli morbidi e fermare (figure 17-18) • Spruzzare per una buona tenuta (figura 19) • Dividere la zona anteriore in due parti, legare un nodo, formando dei riccioli morbidi con le punte e fermare (figure 20-24)

• Créez une section triangulaire de 6 cm de largeur sur le haut de la tête et sur le point le plus en relief à l'arrière de la tête (fig. 2) • Enroulez bien pour créer une base et épinglez, en laissant la queue en dehors (fig.2-3) • Séparez la section supérieure et demandez au client de la maintenir (fig. 4) • Séparez la section latérale et brossez du côté opposé à la base et épinglez dans la base. Répétez la procédure de l'autre côté (fig. 5-8) • Répétez la procédure plusieurs fois de manière à créer un motif en croisillons (fig. 9-11) • Continuez derrière l'oreille en prenant toujours des sections à 45 degrés (fig. 12-16) • Prenez les queues et créez des spires lâches et épinglez (fig. 17-18) • Vaporisez pour maintenir en place (fig.19) • Divisez la partie supérieure en deux, faites un nœud et laissez les queues former des spires sur la partie supérieure et épinglez (fig. 20-24)

• Crear una sección triangular de 6 cm a través de la coronilla en el punto más prominente de la parte posterior de la cabeza. (Fig. 2) • Enrollar bien apretado para crear la base y sujetar con clips, dejando la punta suelta. (Fig.2-3) • Separar la parte superior y pedir a la clienta que la aguante. (Fig. 4) • Separar una sección lateral y cepillar hacia la parte opuesta de la base, sujetándola a la base con clips. Repetir en el otro lado. (Fig. 5-8) • Repetir este proceso varias veces, creando un dibujo entrecruzado. (Fig. 9-11) • Continuar detrás de la oreja, tomando siempre secciones con un ángulo de 45 grados. (Fig. 12-16) • Tomar las puntas y crear remolinos sueltos, sujetándolos con clips. (Fig. 17-18) • Aplicar laca para que se mantenga. (Fig.19) • Separar la parte superior en dos, atar en un nudo, dejando que las puntas se arremolinen en la parte superior, y sujetar con clips. (Fig. 20-24)

• クラウンの上に三角形のセクションを作る（最も尖った角を後頭部に作る）。(図2) • きつくツイストしてベースを作りピンで留める。テールは出しておく。(図2-3) • トップを分け、クライアントにもってもらう。(図4) • サイドをすじ分けし、ベースの反対側へブラッシングしてベースの中にピンで留める。反対側も同様に繰り返す。(図5-8) • 繰り返し行い、十字模様を作る。(図9-11) • 45度の角度ですじ分けをしながら、耳の後ろも行う。(図12-16) • テールをもち、渦巻をゆるく作って、ピンで留める(図17-18)。 • スプレーで固める。(図19) • トップを二つに分け、結ぶ。トップでテールを渦巻かせてピンで留める。(図20-24)

• 在头顶建立一个6厘米三角，尖点在头后面(图2) • 紧紧地编形成发基，夹住，留出发尾(图2-3) • 分出头顶一片头发，让客户拿着(图4) • 分出旁边头发，向发基反方向梳，夹入发基。重复另外一边的头发(图5-8) • 不断重复以形成一个十字图案(图9-11) • 继续耳后头发，45度角处理(图12-16) • 取发稍，做成疏松卷曲，夹住(图17-18) • 喷胶定型(图19) • 头顶头发分两部份，扎成结，发梢在顶部卷曲，夹住(图20-24)

• شكّل خصلة مثلثة الشكل بعرض ٦ سم عبر ذروة الرأس بحيث تكون زاوية المثلث مواجهة نحو القسم الخلفي من الرأس (الصورة ٢) • إفتل الشعر بشدة لتكوين القاعدة وثبتها بدبابيس مع ترك الذيل حر (الصورتين ٢ و٣) • قسّم الشعر الأمامي الى خصل وإطلب من صا حبة الشعر مسكها (الصورة ٤) • خذ خصلة جانبية منها ومشطها نحو الجانب المعاكس للقاعدة وثبتها فيها بدبابيس. كرر نفس العملية على الجهة الأخرى من الرأس (الصور ٥ الى ٨) • كرر هذه العملية مرة بعد مرة لخلق نمط متشابك (الصور ٩ الى ١١) • تابع هذا الإجراء وراء الأذن بحيث تلتقط دائماً خصل مائلة بزاوية ٤٥ (الصور ١٢ الى ١٦) • إلتقط الذيول وشكّل بها لفائف مستديرة غير مشدودة مع ربطها بدبابيس (الصورتين ١٧ و١٨) • رش الشعر لتثبيت التسريحة (الصورة ١٩) • إقسم المسا حة العليا من الشعر الى قسمين وإربطهما على شكل عقدة وأترك الأطراف تلتف   حول أعلى الرأس وأربطها بدبابيس (الصور ٢٠ الى ٢٤)

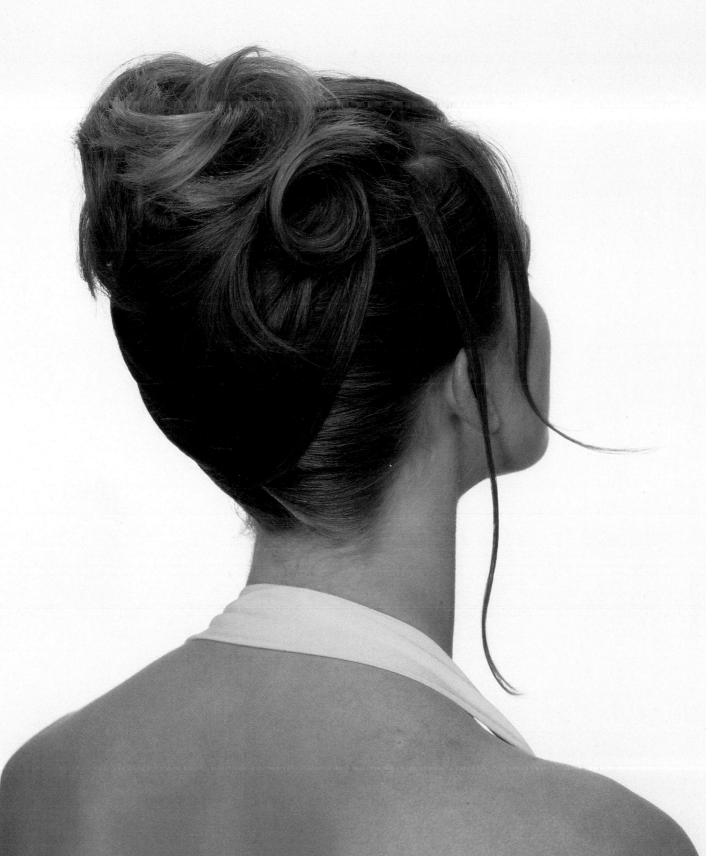

WHITE LILLIES

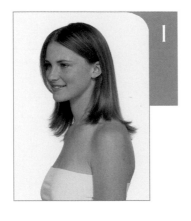

1

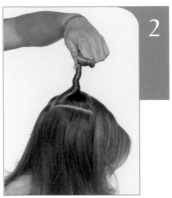

2

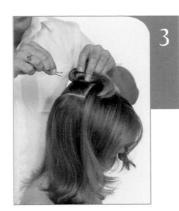

3

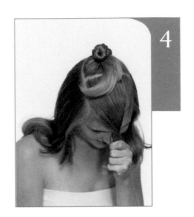

4

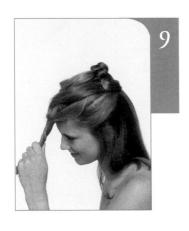

9

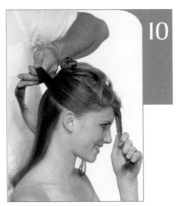

10

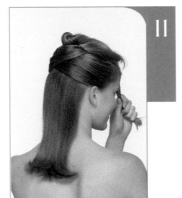

11

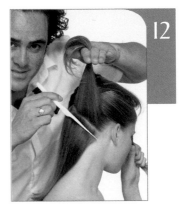

12

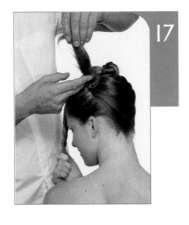

17

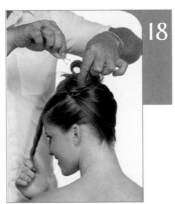

18

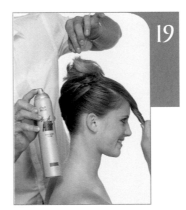

19

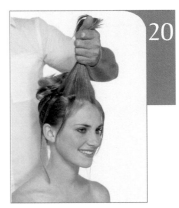

20

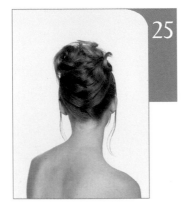

25

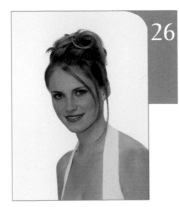

26

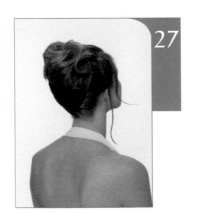

27

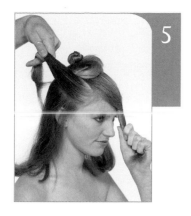
5

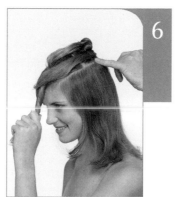
6

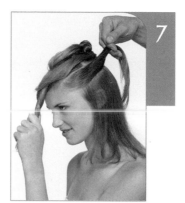
7

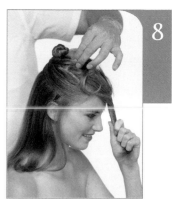
8

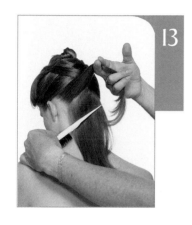
13

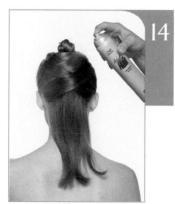
14

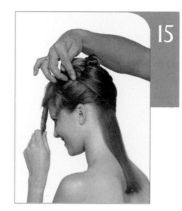
15

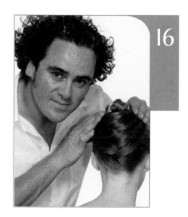
16

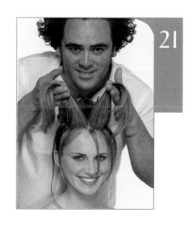
21

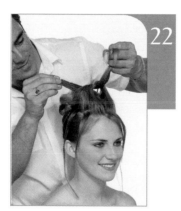
22

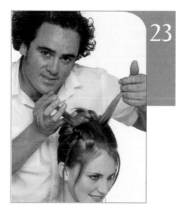
23

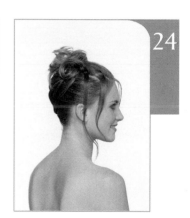
24

WHITE SWAN

• Set hair with hot rollers (fig. 2) • Section from ear to ear and place ponytail into crown area (fig. 3) • Backcomb ponytail and cover with hairnet. Twist surplus hairnet and pin to base (fig. 4-7) • Pin into a firm crescent shape (fig. 8) • Take a section and treat with product (fig. 9) • Create waves with hair, lay onto base and pin. Repeat until base is covered. (fig. 10-22) • Wrap front section around face to soften (fig. 23)

• Haare auf heißen Lockenwicklern aufrollen (Abb. 2) • Haare von Ohr zu Ohr abtrennen und den Pferdeschwanz in den Scheitelbereich bringen (Abb. 3) • Den Pferdeschwanz toupieren und mit einem Haarnetz abdecken. Überschüssiges Haarnetz drehen und am Unterhaar feststecken (Abb. 4-7) • Halbmondförmig feststecken (Abb. 8) • Auf eine Haarsträhne Gel/Mousse geben (Abb. 9) • Das Haar wellenförmig anordnen und auf dem Unterhaar feststecken. Vorgang wiederholen, bis das Unterhaar abgedeckt ist (Abb. 10-22) • Die vorderen Strähnchen so um das Gesicht drapieren, dass sie dem Gesicht weiche Züge verleihen (Abb. 23)

• Mettere in piega i capelli con i bigodini caldi (figura 2) • Dividere da orecchio a orecchio e fare una coda sulla sommita' del capo (figura 3) • Cotonare la coda e coprirla con una retina . Attorcigliare l'eccesso di retina e fermare sulla base (figure 4-7) • Dare forma a una mezzaluna e fermare (figura 8) • Prendere una ciocca e applicare il prodotto (figura 9) • Creare onde con la ciocca e fermare sulla base. Ripetere fino ad avere coperto l'intera base (figure 10-22) • La sezione anteriore incornicia il viso in maniera morbida (figura 23)

• Traitez les cheveux aux rouleaux à chaud (fig. 2) • Séparez d'une oreille à l'autre et placez une queue de cheval sur le haut de la tête (fig. 3) • Peignez la queue de cheval en arrière et couvrez d'un filet à cheveux. Enroulez le filet en excès et épinglez sur la base (fig. 4-7) • Epinglez de manière à former une forme en croissant solide (fig. 8) • Prenez une section et traitez au produit (fig. 9) • Créez une ondulation avec les cheveux, placez sur la base et épinglez. Répétez la procédure jusqu'à ce que la base soit couverte. (fig. 10-22) • Roulez la section avant autour du visage pour adoucir (fig. 23)

• Colocar rulos calientes en el cabello. (Fig. 2) • Separar una sección de oreja a oreja y hacer una cola en la parte de la coronilla. (Fig. 3) • Peinar la cola hacia atrás y cubrir con el postizo. Enrollar el postizo sobrante y sujetar a la base con un clip. (Fig. 4-7) • Formar una media luna sujetando con clips. (Fig. 8) • Tomar una sección del cabello y aplicar producto. (Fig. 9) • Crear ondas con el cabello, colocar sobre la base y sujetar con clips. Repetir hasta cubrir toda la base. (Fig. 10-22) • Enmarcar la cara con la parte frontal del cabello para suavizar la expresión. (Fig. 23)

• ホットローラーでヘアをセットする。（図2） • 耳から耳にかけて分け、クラウンにポニーテールを作る。（図3） • バックコームでポニーテールに逆毛をたて、ヘアネットで覆う。余分なヘアネットはツイストして、ベースにピンで留める。（図4-7） • 三日月の形にしてきつくピンで留める。（図8） • 一すじとり、トリートメント剤で整える。（図9） • ヘアで波を作り、ベースの上にもってきてピンで留める。ベースがカバーされるまで、同様に繰り返す。（図10-22） • フロントをフェースの周りに巻き付けてやわらかい感じをだす。（図23）

• 用热卷发筒处理头发(图2) • 从耳到耳分离头发，在头顶出扎马尾(图3) • 逆梳马尾，用发网盖住，绞剩余发网，夹入发基(图4-7) • 夹成一个结实的弯月状(图8) • 取一部份头发，用发剂处理(图9) • 头发做成波浪，置于发基上，夹住。重复至覆盖发基。(图10-22) • 让前发贴住脸，成温柔效果(图23)

• صفف الشعر على لفائف مسخنة كهربائياً (الصورة ٢) • قسّم الشعر الى خصل من الأذن الى الأذن وشكّل ما تبقى من الشعر بذيل فرس في ذروة الرأس (الصورة ٣) • مشّط ذيل الفرس بالإتجاه العكسي ثم ضع شبكة شعر عليه . لف القسم الزائد من الشبكة وإربطه الى القاعدة بدبابيس (الصور ٤ الى ٧) • صفف ذيل الفرس على شكل هلال مستخدماً دبابيس (الصورة ٨) • ضع منتج التصفيف على خصلة من الهلال (الصورة ٩) • صفف الشعر على شكل أمواج وأرخه على القاعدة مع تثبيته بدبابيس. كرر الإجراء الى أن تغطي القاعدة بكاملها (الصور ١٠ الى ٢٢) • إسدل القسم الأمامي من الشعر حول الوجه لتلطيف التسريحة (الصورة ٢٣)

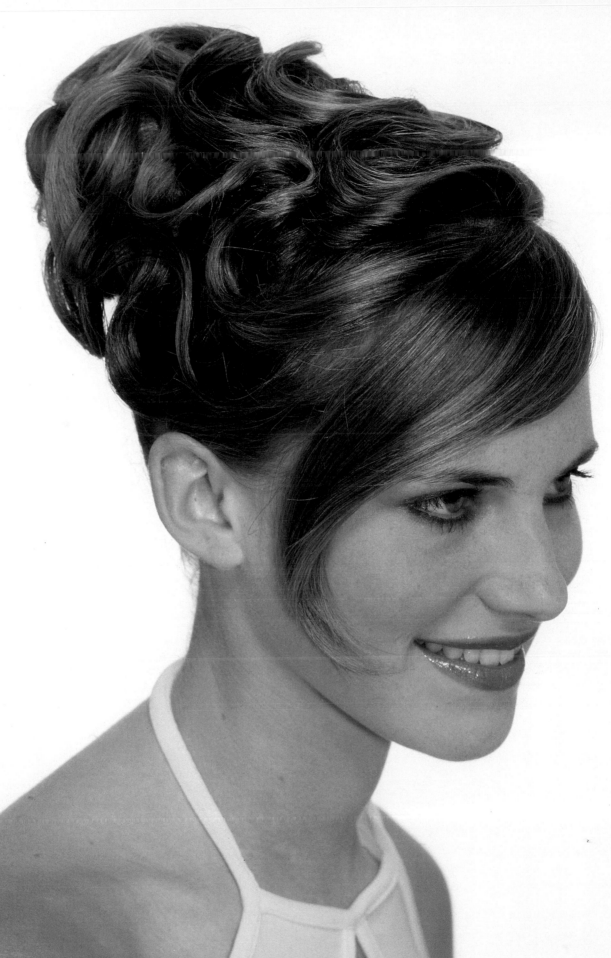

WHITE SWAN

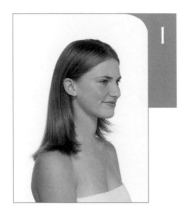

1

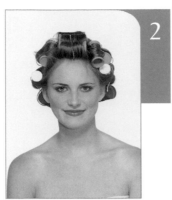

2

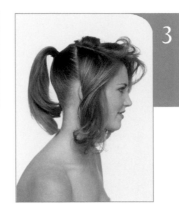

3

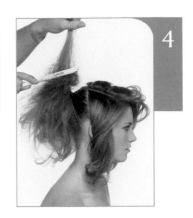

4

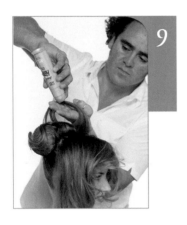

9

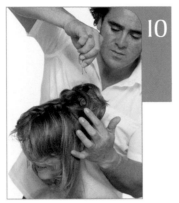

10

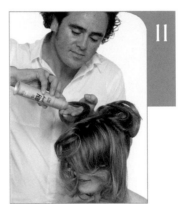

11

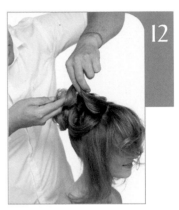

12

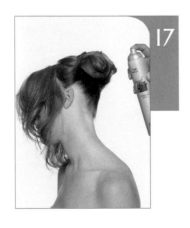

17

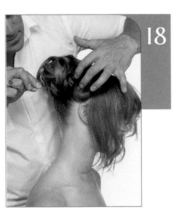

18

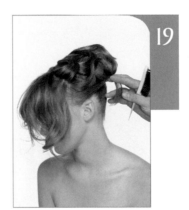

19

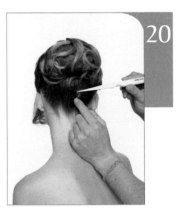

20

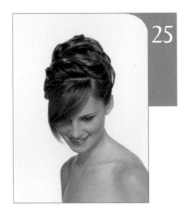

25

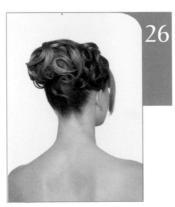

26

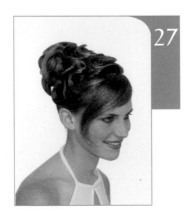

27

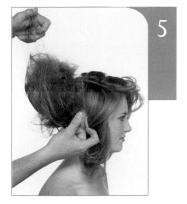

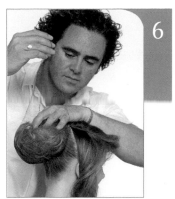

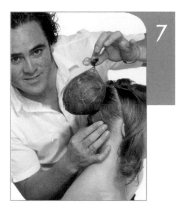

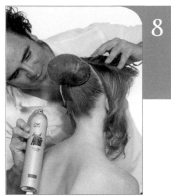

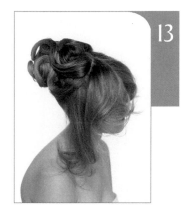

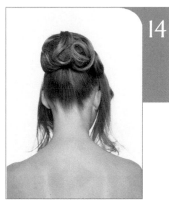

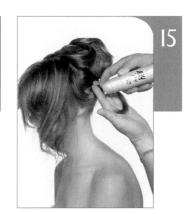

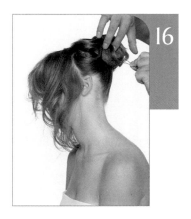

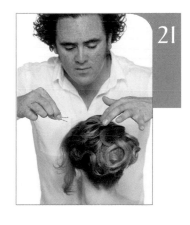

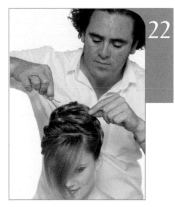

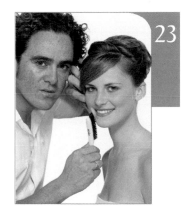

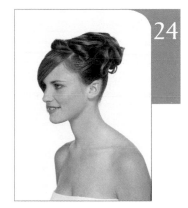

WHITE CHRISTMAS

 • Create base by sectioning 2cm above hairline and place into ponytail (fig. 1-2) • Twist ponytail into two sections and pin (fig. 3-5) • Backcomb tails and spray (fig. 6-7) • Pull ends toward neck and pin (fig. 8-9) • Cross over side back sections and pin (fig. 10-11) • Place styling product into front area. Take strands from both sides and allow to criss-cross over top and base. Pin and spray. (fig. 12-21)

 • Für das Unterhaar 2 cm oberhalb der Haarlinie abtrennen und zu einem Pferdeschwanz binden (Abb. 1-2) • Den Pferdeschwanz in zwei Abschnitte drehen und feststecken (Abb. 3-5) • Die Spitzen toupieren und mit Haarspray in Form sprühen (Abb. 6-7) • Die Enden zum Nacken ziehen und feststecken (Abb. 8-9) • Die rückwärtigen seitlichen Haarabschnitte überkreuzen und feststecken (Abb. 10-11) • Auf die Haare vorne Gel/Mousse geben. Die Strähnen von beiden Seiten nehmen und über das Ober- und Unterhaar kreuzen lassen. Feststecken und mit Haarspray in Form sprühen (Abb. 12-21)

 • Creare la base separando 2cm al di sopra dell'attaccatura e fare una coda (figure 1-2) • Attorcigliare la coda in due sezioni e fermare (figure 3-5) • Cotonare le code e spruzzare (figure 6-7) • Tirare le punte verso la nuca e fermare (figure 8-9) • Incrociare le ciocche e fermare (figure 10-11) • Applicare il prodotto nella zona anteriore. Prendere delle ciocche da entrambi i lati e incrociarle sulla parte superiore e sulla base. Fermare e spruzzare (figure 12-21)

 • Créez une base en séparant les cheveux à 2cm au-dessus des racines et mettez en queue de cheval (fig. 1-2) • Enroulez la queue de cheval en deux sections et épinglez (fig. 3-5) • Peignez les queues en arrière et vaporisez (fig. 6-7) • Tirez les extrémités vers le cou et épinglez (fig. 8-9) • Croisez les sections latérales et épinglez (fig. 10-11) • Appliquez le produit de coiffure sur la section avant. Prenez des mèches des deux côtés et croisez par-dessus le haut et la base. Epinglez et vaporisez. (fig. 12-21)

 • Crear la base separando una sección 2 cm. por encima de la línea del cabello y poner en una cola. (Fig. 1-2) • Enrollar la cola en dos secciones y sujetar con clips. (Fig. 3-5) • Peinar las colas hacia atrás y rociar con laca. (Fig. 6-7) • Tirar de las puntas hacia el cuello y sujetar con clips. (Fig. 8-9) • Cruzar las secciones laterales posterior y sujetar con clips. (Fig. 10-11) • Aplicar producto moldeador en la parte frontal. Tomar hebras de cabello de ambos lados y dejar que se entrelace sobre la base y sobre la parte superior. Sujetar con clips y rociar con laca. (Fig. 12-21)

 • 生え際の上2cmのところで分けてベースを作る。ポニーテールを作る。(図1-2) • ポニーテールをツイストして二つに分け、ピンで留める。(図3-5) • テールをバックコームして逆毛を立てスプレーをかける。(図6-7) • 先端部をネックの方に向けて引っ張り、ピンで留める。(図8-9) • サイドバックを交差させてピンで留める。(図10-11) • フロントをスタイリング剤で整える。両側から束をとり、トップとベースの上で十字形を作る。ピンで留め、スプレーをかける。(図12-21)

 • 头线上2厘米处做成发基，扎成马尾(图1-2) • 编马尾成两部份，夹住(图3-5) • 逆梳发梢，喷胶(图6-7) • 末端拉向颈部，夹住(图8-9) • 交叉后面头发，夹住(图10-11) • 用定型发剂处理前发。两边取发缕，交叉十字于顶部和发基。夹住并喷胶。(图12-21)

• كوّن القاعدة عن طريق تقسيم الشعر وراء حد الجبين بمسافة ٢ سم وأربطه كذيل فرس (الصورتين ١ و٢) • لف ذيل الفرس لتقسيمه الى جزئين وثبته بدبابيس (الصور ٣ الى ٥) • مشّط طرف ذيل الفرس بالإتجاه المعاكس ورشه (الصورتين ٦ و٧) • لف الطرف بإتجاه العنق وثبته بالدبابيس (الصورتين ٨ و٩) • ضع القسمين الجانبيين الخلفيين من الشعر فوق ذروة الرأس وثبتهما بدبابيس (الصورتين ١٠ و١١) • ضع منتج التصفيف على القسم الأمامي من الشعر. التقط خصل من الجانبين ودعها تتشابك فوق ذروة الرأس والقاعدة التي تم تشكيلها أعلاه. ثبتها بالدبابيس ورشها (الصور ١٢ الى ٢١)

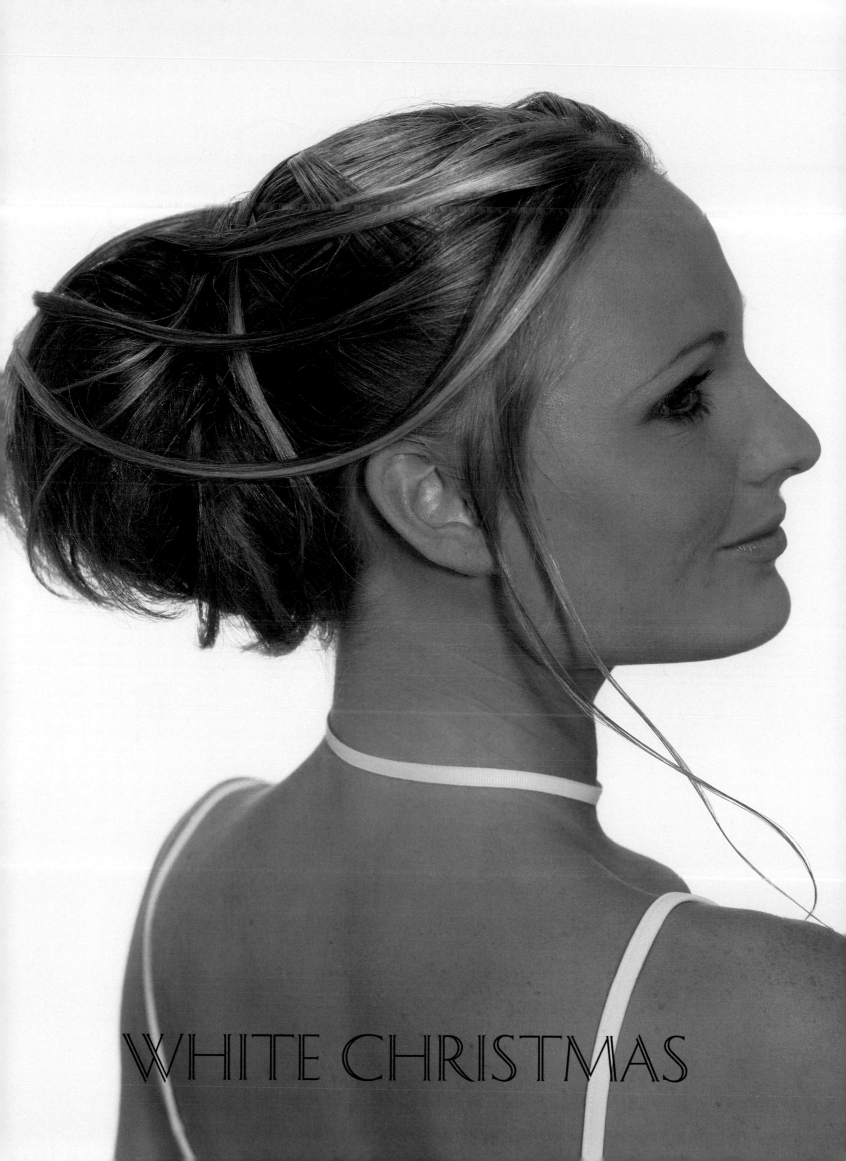

WHITE CHRISTMAS

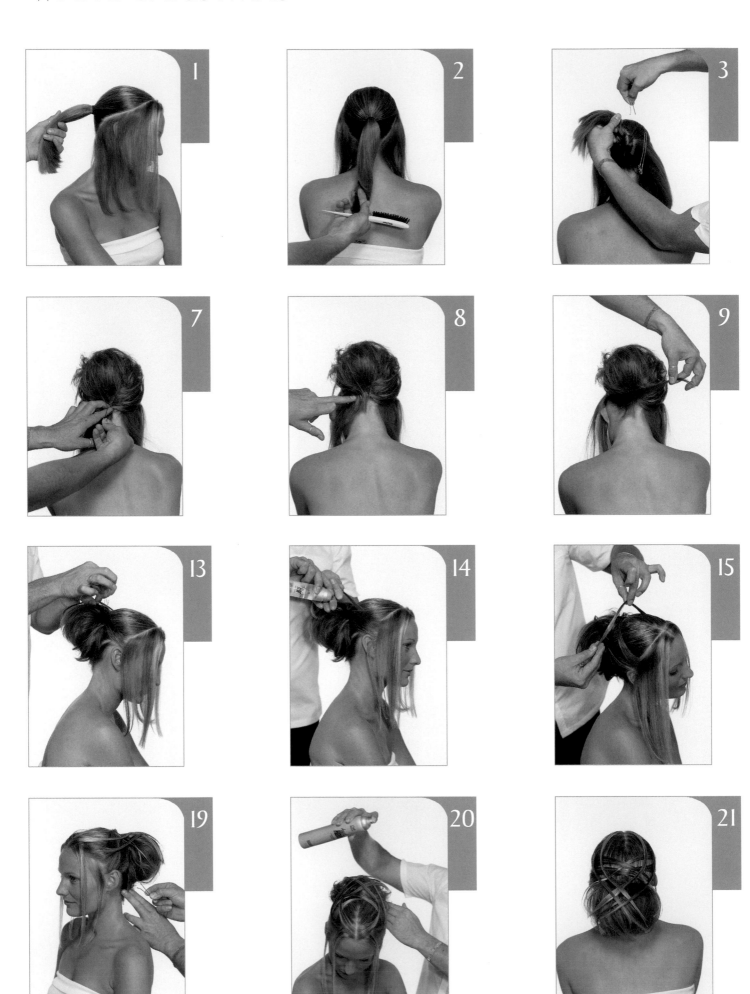

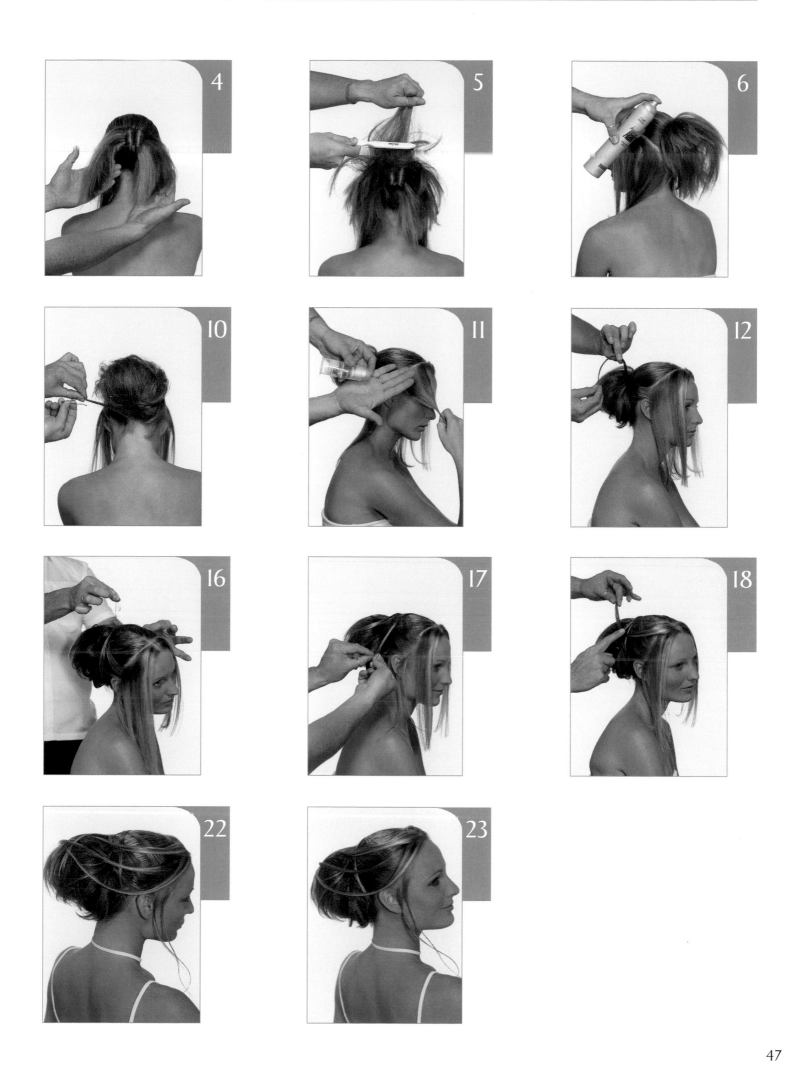

WHITE DOVE

• Place top section into ponytail at crown leaving sides out (fig. 1-2) • Twist side strand over top and twist in tight to scalp with strand from opposite side (fig. 3-4) • Repeat over and over creating a lattice pattern and pin final twist (fig. 5-8) • Sweep sides back and pin into ponytail base (fig. 9-10) • Twist all of remaining back area up and pin into ponytail base (fig. 11) • Pin and spray to create a full back area (fig. 12-13) • Accessorise with small flowers (fig. 14-16)

• Das Oberhaar am Scheitel zu einem Pferdeschwanz binden, dabei jedoch die Seiten auslassen (Abb. 1-2) • Den seitlichen Strang über den Kopf drehen und ihn fest mit dem gegenüberliegenden Strang am Schädel verzwirbeln (Abb. 3-4) • Vorgang wiederholen, bis ein Gittermuster entsteht, dann feststecken (Abb. 5-8) • Seitliche Haare nach hinten kämmen und am Ansatz des Pferdeschwanzes feststecken (Abb. 9-10) • Das übrige Haar verzwirbeln und hoch am Ansatz des Pferdeschwanzes feststecken (Abb. 11) • Feststecken und mit Haarspray in Form sprühen, damit das Ganze Fülle bekommt (Abb. 12-13) • Mit kleinen Blüten schmücken (Abb. 14-16)

Fare una coda sulla sommita' escludendo i capelli dei lati (figure 1-2) • Attorcigliare una ciocca della zona laterale sulla zona superiore e unire attorcigliando una ciocca del lato opposto (figure 3-4) • Ripetere piu' volte per creare un motivo a incrocio e fermare la ciocca finale (figure 5-8) • Tirare i lati indietro e fermarli sulla base (figura 11) • Fermare e spruzzare per completare la parte posteriore (figure 12-14) • Decorare con dei piccoli fiori (figure 14-16)

• Tressez la section supérieure en queue de cheval sur le haut de la tête sans toucher les côtés (fig. 1-2) • Enroulez une mèche latérale sur le dessus et enroulez en serrant contre le cuir chevelu avec la mèche du côté opposé (fig. 3-4) • Répétez la procédure plusieurs fois de manière à créer un motif en croisillons et épinglez la dernière mèche tordue (fig. 5-8) • Tirez les côtés vers l'arrière et maintenez-les et épinglez dans la base de la queue de cheval (fig. 9-10) • Enroulez tout ce qui reste dans la section arrière et épinglez dans la base de la queue de cheval (fig. 11) • Maintenez à l'aide d'une épingle et vaporisez pour volumiser la section arrière (fig. 12-13) • Décorez à l'aide de petites fleurs (fig. 14-16)

• Colocar la sección superior en una cola en la coronilla dejando fuera los lados. (Fig. 1-2) • Enrollar un mechón lateral sobre la parte superior y enrollar de manera apretada con un mechón del lado opuesto. (Fig. 3-4) • Repetir varias veces creando una especie de enrejado y sujetar el bucle final con clips. (Fig. 5-8) • Peinar los lados hacia atrás y sujetar con clips a la base de la cola. (Fig. 9-10) • Enrollar todo el cabello restante de la parte posterior y sujetar con clips en la base de la cola. (Fig. 11) • Sujetar con clips y rociar con laca para crear toda un área posterior. (Fig. 12-13) • Adornar con pequeñas flores. (Fig. 14-16)

• クラウンでトップヘアをポニーテールにする。サイドは外に出しておく。(図1-2) • サイド束をトップでツイストする。反対側の束といっしょに頭皮にきつくツイストする。(図3-4) • 繰り返して格子形を作る。最後のツイストをピンで留める。(図5-8) • サイドはバックへ流してポニーテール・ベースの中にピンで留める。(図9-10) • バックの残りの部分をすべてツイストして持ち上げ、ポニーテール・ベースの中にピンで留める。(図11) • ピンで留め、スプレーをかけてフルバックを作る。(図12-13) • 小さい花で飾る。(図14-16)

• 头顶头发做成马尾，留住边(图1-2) • 编边发(图3-4) • 重复以形成格子图案，夹住(图5-8) • 向后披边发，夹到马尾发根(图9-10) • 将所有后面头发编结，夹入马尾发根(图11) • 夹住并喷胶，形成一个完整的后发区(图12-13) • 以小花朵点缀(图14-16)

• صفف القسم العلوي من الشعر كذيل الفرس وأترك الجانبين سائبين (الصورتين ١ و٢) • إفتل خصلة جانبية فوق أعلى الرأس ثم إفتلها مع خصلة من الجانب الآخر بشدة بحيث تكون ملتصقة مع فروة الرأس (الصورتين ٣ و٤) • كرر هذا الإجراء مرة أخرى لتكوّن نمط متشابك مع تثبيت اللفة الأخيرة بدبابيس (الصور ٥ الى ٨) • إسحب الشعر الجانبي نحو الخلف وثبته بدبابيس الى قاعدة ذيل الفرس (الصورتين ٩ و١٠) • إفتل بقية الشعر الموجود في مؤخرة الرأس وثبته بدبابيس الى قاعدة ذيل الفرس (الصورة ١١) • إشبك القسم الخلفي من التسريحة بدبابيس إضافية مع رشها في نفس الوقت لزيادة حجم التسريحة (الصورتين ١٢ و١٣) • زيّن التسريحة بواسطة زهور صغيرة (الصور ١٤ الى ١٦)

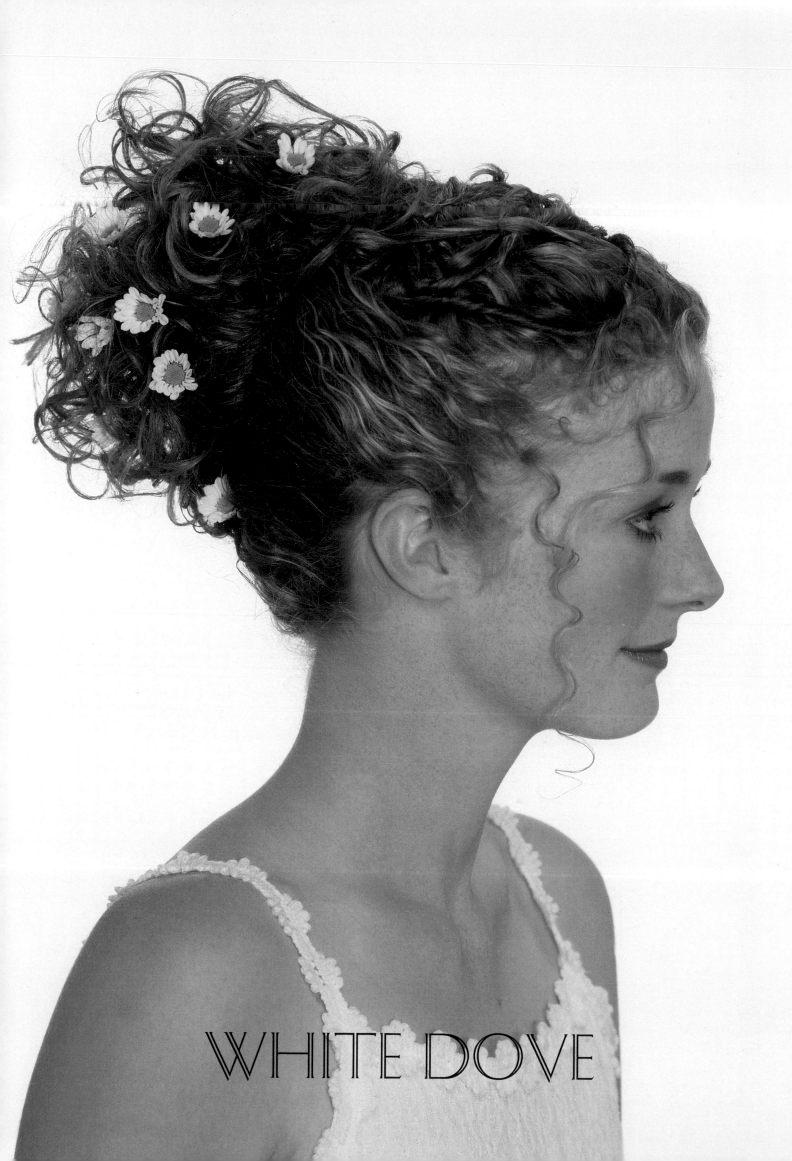

WHITE DOVE

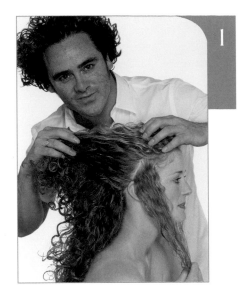

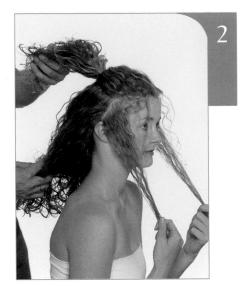

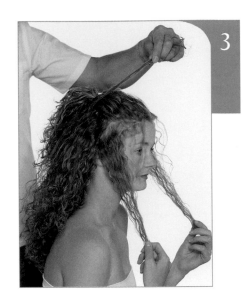

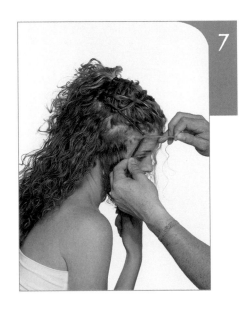

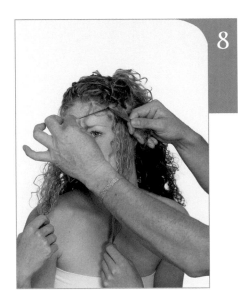

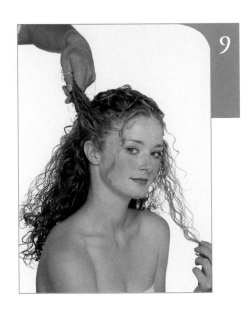

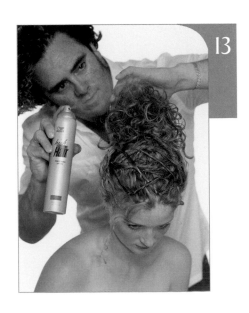

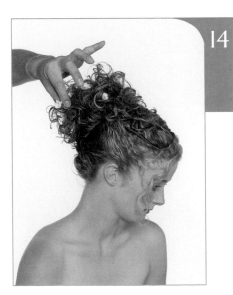

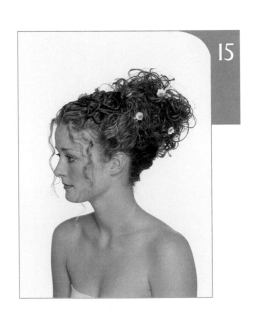

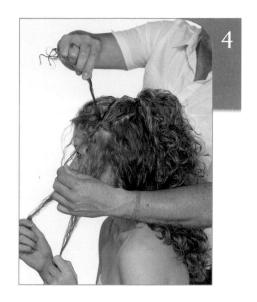

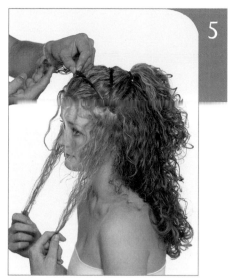

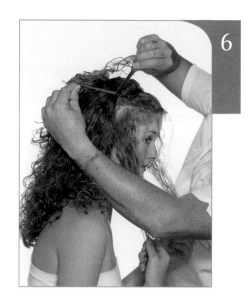

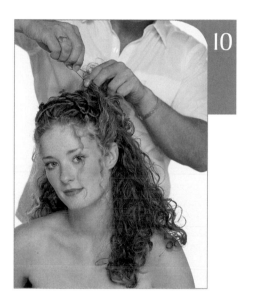

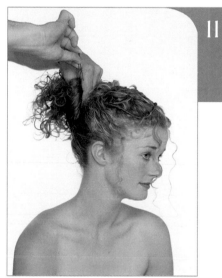

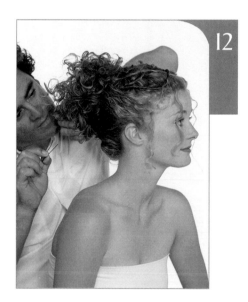

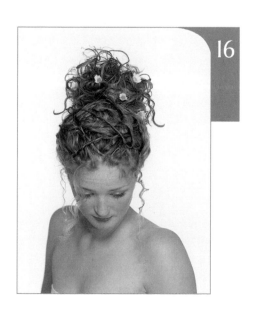

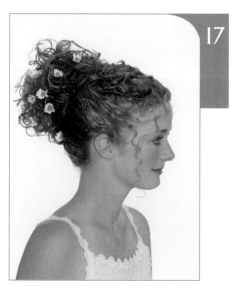

WHITE SATIN

• Set in hot rollers for movement (fig. 1-2) • Divide hair in middle (fig. 4) • Take a section at a 45 degree angle, twist under loosely and pin (fig. 5-6) • Repeat down the side (fig. 7-10) • Place a line of pins at scalp and brush hair away (fig.11) • Repeat down opposite side (fig. 12) • Pinch together and pin bottom two twists (fig. 13-14) • Lift tails, place ribbon and tie on top (fig.15-16) • Backcomb to give volume and shape (fig. 17-18) • Drape and place front section over back area and spray to hold (fig. 19-20)

• Haare auf heißen Lockenwicklern aufwickeln (Abb. 1-2) • Mittelscheitel ziehen (Abb. 4) • Einen Haarabschnitt in einem 45°-Winkel lose drehen und feststecken (Abb. 5-6) • Vorgang auf der anderen Seite wiederholen (Abb. 7-10) • Nadeln an der Kopfhaut anbringen und das Haar wegbürsten (Abb. 11) • Vorgang auf der anderen Seite wiederholen (Abb. 12) • Zusammendrücken und die beiden unteren gedrehten Strähnen feststecken (Abb. 13-14) • Spitzen hochheben, das Band anbringen und oben befestigen (Abb. 15-16) • Die Haare toupieren, um ihnen mehr Volumen und Form zu verleihen (Abb. 17-18) • Drapieren und die Haare vorne über die Haare hinten legen und mit Haarspray in Form sprühen (Abb. 19-20)

• Mettere in piega con bigodini caldi per dare movimento (figure 1-2) • Dividere i capelli al centro (figura 4) • Prendere una sezione diagonale a 45 gradi, attorcigliare in senso orario morbidamente e fermare (figure 5-6) • Ripetere nella zona laterale (figure 7-10) • Fare una linea di forcine e spazzolare i capelli verso l'esterno (figura 11) • Ripetere sul lato opposto (figura 12) • Unire e fermare le due ciocche attorcigliate (figure 13-14) • Sollevare le code, mettere un nastro e legare in alto (figure 15-16) • Cotonare per dare volume e forma (figure 17-18) • Disporre e mettere la sezione anteriore sopra la zona posteriore e spruzzare per tenere in posizione (figure 19-20)

• Traitez avec des rouleaux chauds pour onduler (fig. 1-2) • Divisez les cheveux dans le milieu (fig. 4) • Prenez une section selon un angle de 45 degrés, pliez par-dessous de manière lâche et maintenez à l'aide d'une épingle (fig. 5-6) • Répétez la procédure sur le côté (fig. 7-10) • Placez une ligne d'épingles contre le cuir chevelu et écartez les cheveux à la brosse (fig.11) • Répétez la procédure de l'autre côté (fig. 12) • Pincez ensemble et épinglez les deux spires inférieures (fig. 13-14) • Soulevez les queues, placez le ruban et nouez-le sur le dessus (fig.15-16) • Peignez en arrière pour donner forme et volume (fig. 17-18) • Drapez et placez la section avant sur l'arrière et vaporisez pour maintenir en place (fig. 19-20)

• Colocar rulos calientes para dar movimiento. (Fig. 1-2) • Dividir el cabello por la mitad. (Fig. 4) • Tomar una sección a un ángulo de 45 grados, enrollar dejando un poco suelto y sujetar con clips. (Fig. 5-6) • Repetir al otro lado. (Fig. 7-10) • Colocar una línea de clips en el cuero cabelludo y cepillar el cabello. (Fig.11) • Repetir en el lado opuesto. (Fig. 12) • Unir con los dedos y sujetar con clips los dos bucles inferiores. (Fig. 13-14) • Levantar las colas, colocar una cinta y atar en la parte superior. (Fig.15-16) • Peinar hacia atrás para dar forma y volumen. (Fig. 17-18) • Dejar caer y colocar la sección frontal sobre el área posterior y aplicar laca para que se mantenga. (Fig. 19-20)

• ホットローラーでセットして動きを出す。（図1-2） • 中央でヘアを分ける。（図4） • 45度の角度でセクションをとり、下にゆるくツイストする。ピンで留める。（図5-6） • サイドを下に向けて同様に繰り返す。（図7-10） • 頭皮に一線上にピンを並べ、ブラッシングしてヘアを流す。（図11） • 反対側のサイドも同様に行う。（図12） • 下の二つのツイストをいっしょにつまみ、ピンで留める。（図13-14） • テールを持ち上げ、リボンをトップで結ぶ。（図15-16） • バックコームして逆毛を立て、ボリュームを出し、形を整える。（図17-18） • フロントをバックへ流し、スプレーで固定する。（図19-20）

•设热卷发筒作准备(图1-2) •头发中分(图4) •45度角取一片头发，疏松地扭结，夹住(图5-6) •重复至下面的头发(图7-10) •放一排发卡在头顶，梳理头发(图11) •重复下来至对面(图12) •别在一起，夹住底部两股编结(图13-14) •提起发梢，加发带并扎在顶部(图15-16) •逆梳形成栏状(图17-18) •前发披置在后发区，喷胶定型(图19-20)

• صفف الشعر على لفائف مسخنة كهربائياً لجعله مالساً وسهل الحركة (الصورتين 1 و2) • إقسم الشعر الى قسمين متساويين (الصورة 4) • إلتقط خصلة وشدها بزاوية 45. إفتلها بخفة نحو الداخل وثبتها بدبابيس (الصورتين 5 و6) • كرر هذا الإجراء على إمتداد جانب الرأس (الصورة 12) • إجمع اللفتين السفليتين معاً وثبتهما بدبابيس (الصورتين 13 و14) • إرفع طرفيهما . ضع الشريط وإربطه في أعلى الرأس (الصورتين 15 و16) • مشّط الأطراف بالإتجاه المعاكس لزيادة الحجم وضبط الشكل (الصورتين 17 و18) • إسدل القسم الأمامي من الشعر ومدده بنعومة فوق المسا حة الخلفية ثم رشه للتثبيت (الصورتين 19 و20)

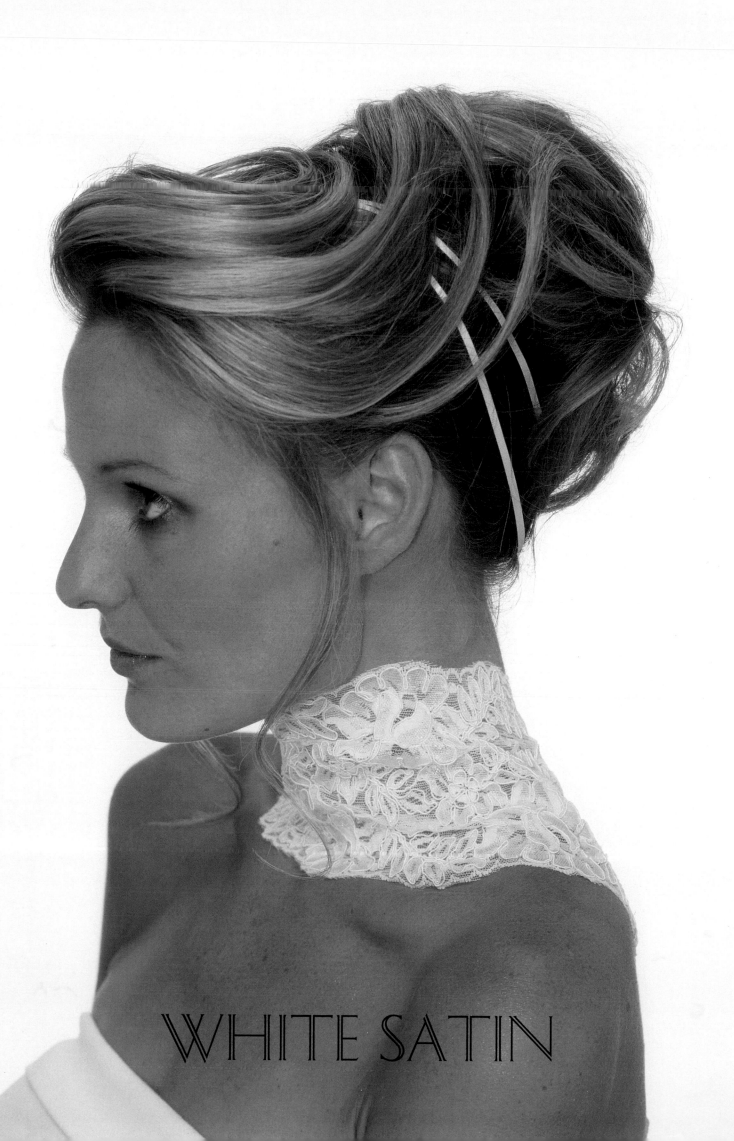

WHITE SATIN

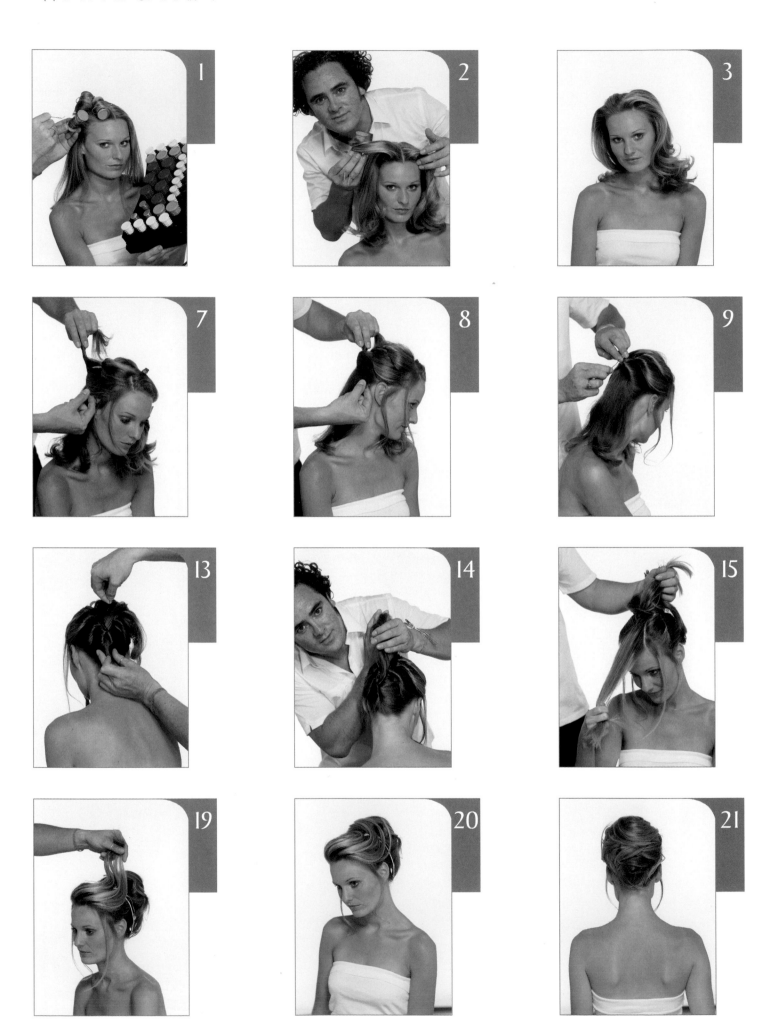

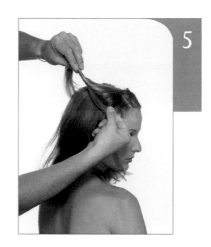

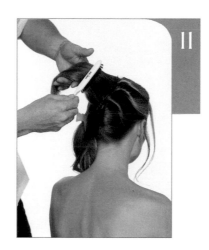

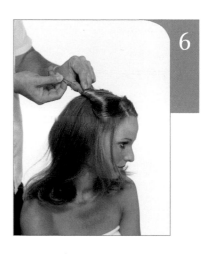

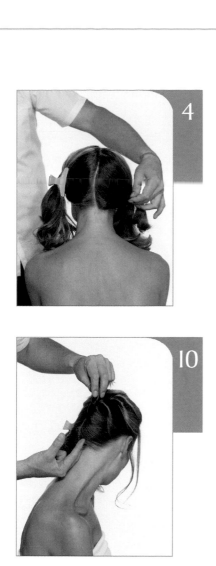

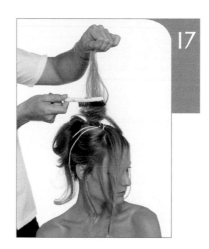

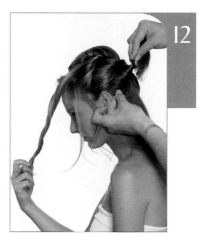

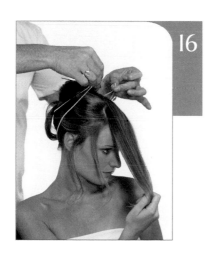

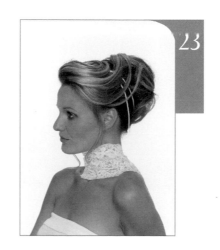

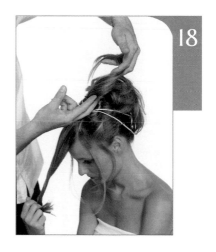

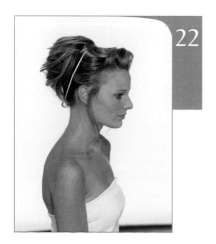

WHITE LINEN

 • Section behind ear to crown to behind ear (fig. 2) • Twist front hair behind ear (both sides) and pin (fig. 3-7) • Take two sections from behind crown (1.5 cm apart) and treat with product (fig. 8) • Take strand from right side and place under middle strands and pin temporarily (fig. 9) • Take 3 strands and place a strand from left side under and pin temporarily (fig. 10-11) • Repeat above 3 steps back and forth creating a basket weave (fig. 12-18) • Split back section into two (fig. 19) • Twist and cross over pinning to either side (fig. 20-21) • Remove temporary pins, take tails of strands and tuck into side twists (fig. 22-25) • Finish by placing tails into fans (fig. 26)

 • Haarabschnitt hinter den Ohren vom Scheitel abtrennen (Abb. 2) • Vordere Haarsträhne auf beiden Seiten drehen und hinter den Ohren feststecken (Abb. 3-7) o Zwei Haarsträhnen von der Scheitelrückseite (Abstand von 1,5 cm) abtrennen und mit Haarspray einsprühen (Abb. 8) •Eine Haarsträhne von rechts unter den mittleren Strähnen durchführen und vorübergehend feststecken (Abb. 9) • Eine Haarsträhne von links unter drei Strähnen durchführen und vorübergehend feststecken (Abb. 10-11) • Diese drei Schritte wiederholen, bis es wie Korbflechterei aussieht (Abb. 12-18) • Haare im Nacken zweiteilen (Abb. 19) • Verdrehen und über Kreuz auf der jeweils gegenüberliegenden Seite feststecken (Abb. 20-21) • Die Behelfsnadeln entfernen und die Strähnchenenden unter den seitlich festgesteckten Zöpfen feststecken (Abb. 22-25) • Abschließend die Strähnen auffächern (Abb. 26)

 • Dividere i capelli da orecchio, sommita', orecchio (figura 2) • Attorcigliare i capelli della zona anteriore (su entrambi i lati) e fermarli (figura 3-7) • Prendere due ciocche dalla sommita' (alla distanza di 1,5 cm) e applicare il prodotto (figura 8) • Prendere una ciocca dal lato destro e passandolo sotto le ciocche centrali e fermate temporaneamente (figura 9) • Prendere tre ciocche facendo passare una ciocca dal lato sinistro sotto e fermate temporaneamente (figure 10-11) • Ripetere i passaggi precedenti piu' volte per creare un intreccio simile a un cestino (figure 12-18) • Dividere la zona posteriore in due (figura 19) • Attorcigliare e incrociare fermando entrambi i lati (figure 20-21) • Rimuovere le forcine temporanee e inserite le ciocche nei capelli attorcigliati laterali (figure 22-25) • Completare formando un ventaglio con le code rimaste (figura 26)

 • Séparez la section de derrière l'oreille au haut de la tête et placez-la derrière l'oreille (fig. 2) • Enroulez les cheveux de devant derrière l'oreille (des deux côtés) et épinglez (fig. 3-7) • Prenez deux sections de derrière le haut de la tête (à 1, 5 cm de distance) et traitez au produit (fig. 8) • Prenez une mèche du côté droit et placez-la sous les mèches du milieu et épinglez temporairement (fig. 9) • Prenez trois mèches et placez une mèche du côté gauche en dessous et épinglez temporairement (fig. 10-11) • Répétez la procédure en 3 étapes ci-dessus de manière à créer un motif en corbeille (fig. 12-18) • Divisez en deux la section arrière (fig. 19) • Enroulez et croisez en épinglant de part et d'autre (fig. 20-21) • Retirez les épingles temporaires, prenez les extrémités des mèches et passez-les sous les spires latérales (fig. 22-25) • Finissez en arrangeant les queues en éventails (fig. 26)

 •Separar una sección desde detrás de la oreja hasta la coronilla. (Fig. 2) • Enrollar el cabello delantero detrás de la oreja (en ambos lados) y sujetar con un clip. (Fig. 3-7) • Tomar dos secciones de detrás de la coronilla (con 1,5 cm de distancia) y aplicar producto. (Fig. 8) • Tomar un mechón de la parte derecha y color debajo de los mechones centrales, sujetándolo temporalmente con un clip. (Fig. 9) • Tomar 3 mechones y colocar un mechón del lado izquierdo por debajo sujetándolo temporalmente con un clip. (Fig. 10-11) • Repetir los 3 pasos anteriores creando una especie de tejido como si fuera rafia. (Fig. 12-18) • Dividir la sección posterior en dos partes. (Fig. 19) • Enrollar y sujetar con clips de forma cruzada a cada lado. (Fig. 20-21) • Retirar los clips temporales, sacar las puntas de los mechones e introducir en las partes enrolladas laterales (Fig. 22-25) • Acabar colocando las puntas en forma de abanico (Fig. 26)

 • 耳の後ろからクラウンにかけて分ける。(図2) • フロントを耳の後ろ(両側)にツイストして、ピンで留める(図3-7)。 • クラウンの後ろから二つのセクションをとり(間隔1.5cm)、トリートメント剤で整える。(図8) • 右側から一束とり、中央の束の下にもってきて、一時的にピンで留める。(図9) • 三束とり、左側の束を下にもってきて、一時的にピンで留める。(図10-11) • 上の三段階を繰り返し、篭織りを作る。(図12-18)。 • バックを二つに分ける。(図19) • ツイストして、交差させる。両側をピンで留める。(図20-21) • 留めておいたピンを取り外し、各束のテールをとって、サイドツイストの中に押し込む。(図22-25) • テールを扇形にして終了。(図26)

 • 耳后到头顶再到耳后的一片头发(图2) • 耳后的前发编结(两边),夹住(图3-7) • 从头顶后取两片头发(间隔1.5厘米),用发剂处理(图8) • 从右边取一缕头置于中间发缕下面,暂用发卡卡住(图9) • 取3缕发,从左边将一缕置于下面,用发卡暂夹住(图10-11) • 前后重复以上3步骤,形成篮子编织(图12-18) • 将后面的头发分成两部份(图19) • 编结并向两边夹住(图20-21) • 将临时发卡拿走,把发缕梢塞入旁边的编结里(图22-25) • 以发尾摆成扁扇状结束(图26)

 • قسّن الشعر الى خصل من وراء الأذن الى ذروة الرأس ومنه الى خلف الأذن الأخرى (الصورة ٢) • أفتل مقدمة الشعر الموجود وراء الأذن (في الجهتين) وثبت الجديلتين بالدبابيس (الصور ٣ الى ٧). • خذ خصلتين من وراء ذروة الرأس (مع فاصل ١،٥ سم بينهما) وضع منتج التصفيف عليهما (الصورة ٨) • إلتقط ضفيرة من الجهة اليمنى وضعها تحت الضفائر الوسطى وثبتهما مؤقتاً بدبابيس (الصورة ٩) • إمسك الضفائر الثلاث وضع ضفيرة من الجهة اليسرى تحتها ثم ثبتهامؤقتا بدبابيس (الصورتان ١٠ و١١) • كرر الخطوات الثلاث أعلاه ذهاباً وإياباً لتكوين ما يشبه حياكة السلة (الصور ١٢ امى ١٨) • إقسم الجزء الخلفي من الشعر الى قسمين (الصورة ١٩) • إفتل القسم الأيمن وضعه فوق الجهة اليسرى ثم إفتل القسم الأيسر وضعه فوق الجهة اليمنى (الصورتين ٢٠ و٢١) • إنزع دبابيس التثبيت المؤقت ثم إلتقط ذيول الضفائر وأدخلها في الضفائر الجانبية (الصور ٢٢ الى ٢٥) • إنهي التسريحة بتسريح الذيول على شكل مراوح.

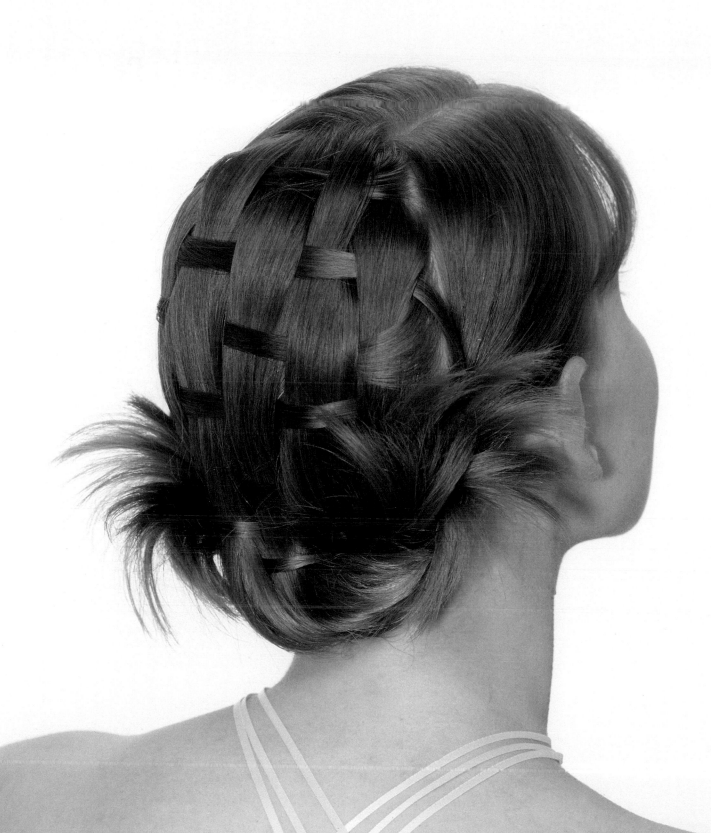

WHITE LINEN

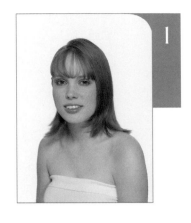

1

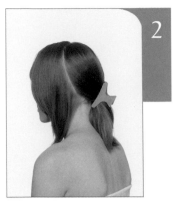

2

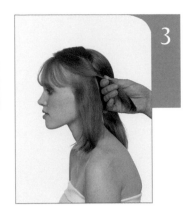

3

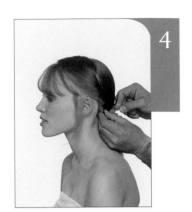

4

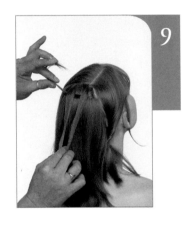

9

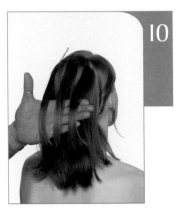

10

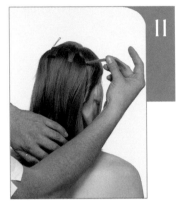

11

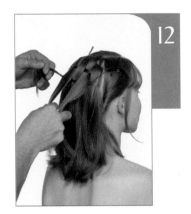

12

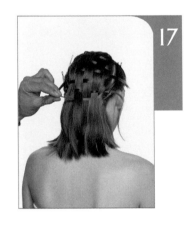

17

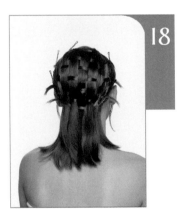

18

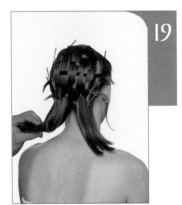

19

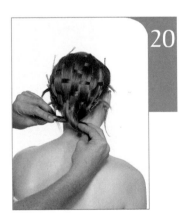

20

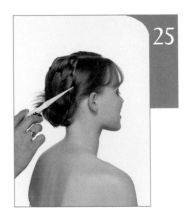

25

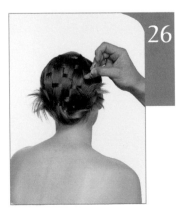

26

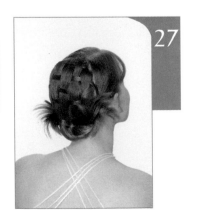

27

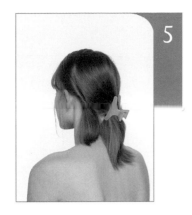

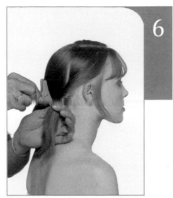

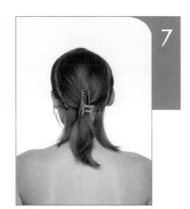

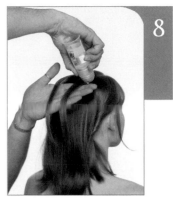

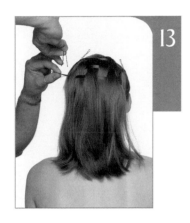

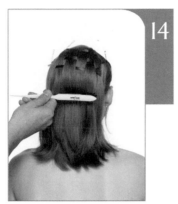

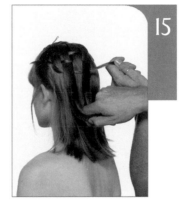

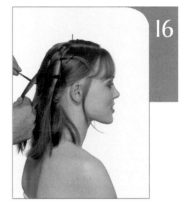

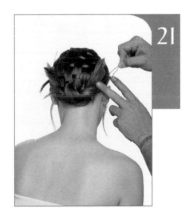

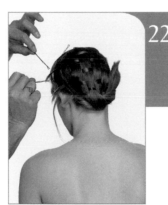

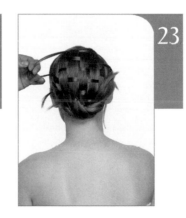

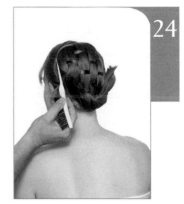

WHITE MISCHIEF

• Section triangle at crown, twisting into a tight base. Pin to hold. (fig. 1-3) • Take a slice from above ear and twist (fig. 4-5) • Holding a fine thread of hair, push twist back towards scalp and pin (fig. 6-9) • Repeat down the back of the head, pinning into the centre (fig. 10-18) • Repeat on the other side (fig. 19-20) • Section front area and repeat process, pinning into base (fig. 21-24) • Spray tails into place (fig. 25) • Style front with tongs for softness (fig. 26-27)

• Ein Dreieck am Scheitel abtrennen und fest als Unterhaar verzwirbeln. Feststecken. (Abb. 1-3) • Eine Strähne von oberhalb des Ohres verdrehen (Abb. 4-5) • Eine feine Haarsträhne nach hinten verzwirbeln und feststecken (Abb. 6-9) • Vorgang im Nacken wiederholen, die Strähnen jeweils in der Mitte feststecken (Abb. 10-18) • Vorgang auf der anderen Seite wiederholen (Abb. 19-20) • Haare vorne teilen und den Vorgang wiederholen, Haare am Unterhaar feststecken (Abb. 21-24) • Spitzen mit Haarspray in Form sprühen (Abb. 25) • Haare vorne mit einem Lockenstab stylen, um einen weicheren Look zu erzielen (Abb. 26-27)

• Dividere un triangolo sulla sommita' del capo, attorcigliare e fermare per creare una base (figure 1-3) • Prendere una ciocca dal lato e attorcigliare (figure 4-5) • Tenendo una piccolissima quantita' di capelli far scivolare la ciocca attorcigliata verso la cute e fermare (figure 6-9) • Ripetere nella parete posteriore fermando al centro (figure 10-18) • Ripetere dal lato opposto (figure 19-20) • Dividere la zona anteriore e ripetere il procedimento fermando alla base (figure 21-24) • Spruzzare le punte per dare definizione (figura 25) • Dare movimento con il ferro arricciapelli nella zona frontale (figure 26-27)

• Séparez un triangle sur le haut de la tête, en enroulant de manière à former une base solide. Maintenez à l'aide d'une épingle. (fig. 1-3) • Prenez une section de cheveux au-dessus de l'oreille et enroulez (fig. 4-5) • En tenant une fine mèche de cheveux, poussez en réenroulant vers le cuir chevelu et épinglez (fig. 6-9) • Répétez la procédure sur l'arrière de la tête, en fixant au centre à l'aide d'une épingle (fig. 10-18) • Répétez la procédure de l'autre côté (fig. 19-20) • Séparez la partie avant et répétez la procédure, en épinglant sur la base (fig. 21-24) • Vaporisez les queues en place (fig. 25) • Coiffez le devant avec des fers pour assurer la douceur du cheveu (fig. 26-27)

• Marcar un triángulo en la coronilla, enrollándolo en una base apretada. Sujetar con clips. (Fig. 1-3) • Tomar una sección del cabello encima de la oreja y enrollar. (Fig. 4-5) • Sujetando una hebra fina de cabello, tirar del bucle hacia atrás hacia el cuero cabelludo y sujetar con un clip. (Fig. 6-9) • Repetir en la parte inferior trasera de la cabeza, sujetándolo con clips en el centro. (Fig. 10-18) • Repetir en el otro lado. (Fig. 19-20) • Dividir la parte delantera y repetir el proceso, sujetando con clips a la base. (Fig. 21-24) • Rociar las puntas con laca para que se aguanten. (Fig. 25) • Adornar la parte delantera con pinzas para aportar suavidad. (Fig. 26-27)

• クラウンに三角形のセクションを作る。きつくツイストしてベースを作る。ピンで固定する。(図1-3) • 耳の上から一すじとってツイストする。(図4-5)。• ヘアを細い束にとり、頭皮に向けてツイストして押す。ピンで留める。(図6-9) • 同様に後頭部を下側へ向けて繰り返す。センターヘピンで留める。(図10-18) • 反対側も同様に行う。(図19-20) • フロントをセクション分けし、同様に行う。ベースにピンで留める。(図21-24) • テールにスプレーをかける。(図25) • トングを使ってフロントをやわらかく整える。(図26-27)

• 头顶三角，绞成一个紧的发基。夹住(图1-3) • 从耳朵上方取一片头发，编结(图4-5) • 握住一缕头发，推编结向头顶，夹住(图6-9) • 重复过程至后发，夹入中央(图10-18) • 另一边重复(图19-20) • 取前发，重复过程，夹如发基(图21-24) • 喷胶于发梢定型(图25) • 用夹子为前发造型(图26-27)

• شكّل قسم من الشعر في ذروة الرأس كمثلث ولفه بشدة لتكوين قاعدة. ثبته بدبابيس (الصور ١ الى ٣) • خذ خصلة شعر فوق الأذن وإفتلها (الصورتين ٤ و٥) • إمسك خيط رفيع من الشعر ثم إدفع الخصلة المفتولة باتجاه فروة الرأس وثبتها بدبابيس (الصور ٦ الى ٩) • كرر هذا الإجراء على إمتداد مؤخرة الرأس مع تثبيت الشعر في الوسط (الصور ١٠ الى ١٨) • كرر نفس الإجراء على جانب الرأس الآخر (الصور ١٨ الى ٢٠) • إقسم الجزء الأمامي من الشعر الى قسمين وكرر نفس العملية مع تثبيت الشعر في القاعدة المذكورة أعلاه (الصور ٢١ الى ٢٤) • رش الذيول لكي تثبتها في موضعها (الصورة ٢٥) • ملّس الشعر الأمامي بواسطة الملقط الساخن لتليينه (الصورتين ٢٦ و٢٧)

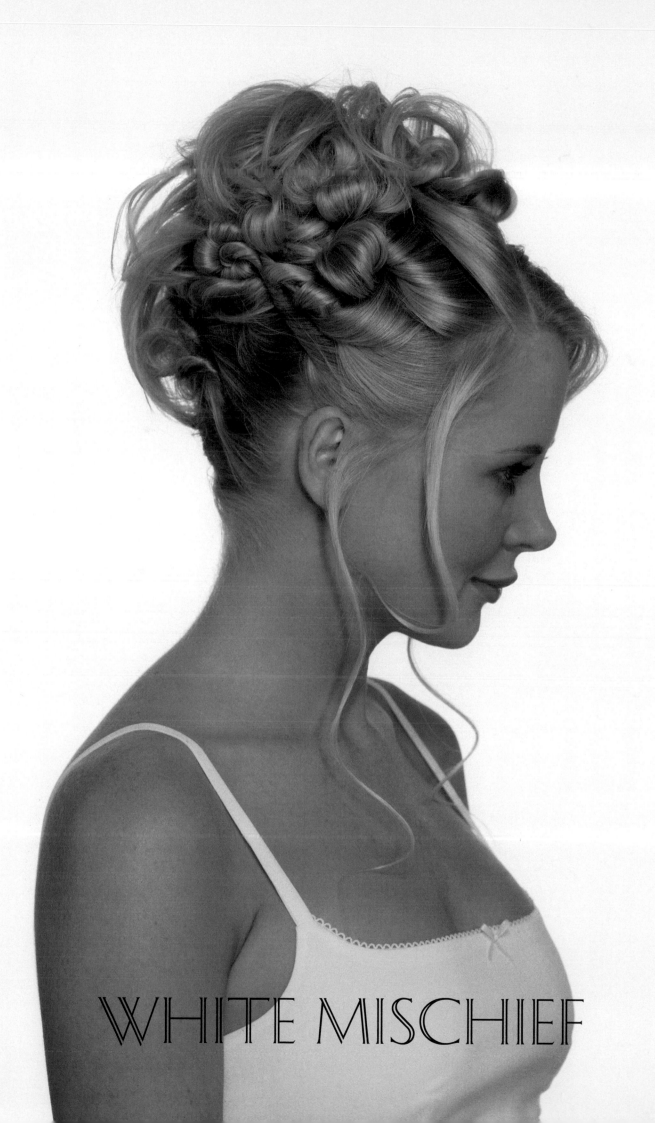

WHITE MISCHIEF

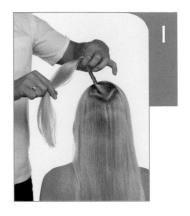

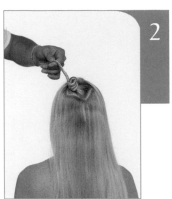

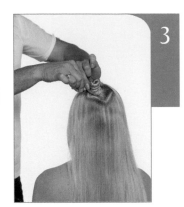

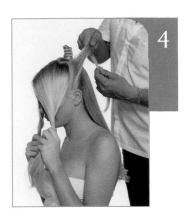

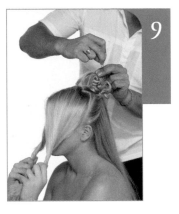

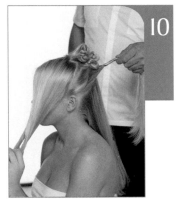

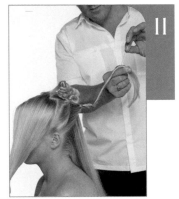

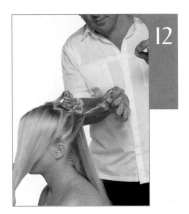

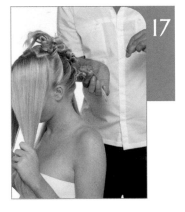

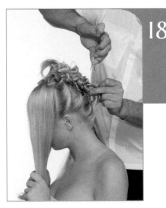

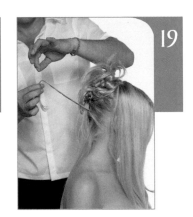

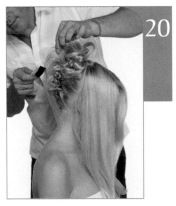

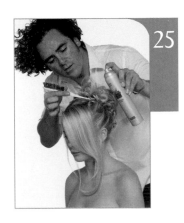

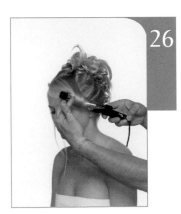

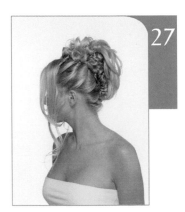

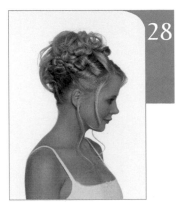

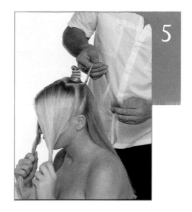

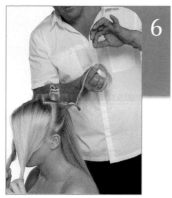

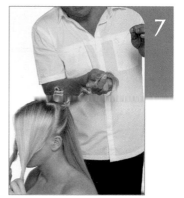

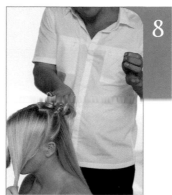

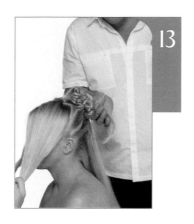

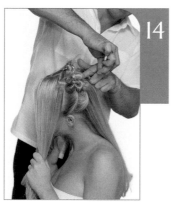

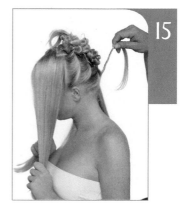

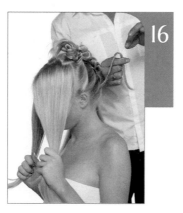

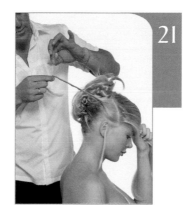

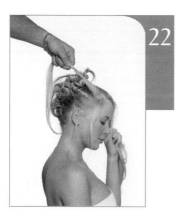

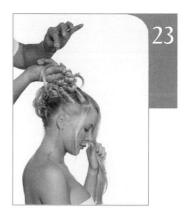

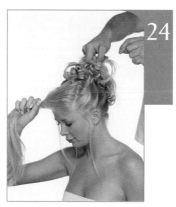

WHITE PORCELAIN

 • Treat with product and blow-dry to straighten (fig. 1-3) • Section back area off and place ponytail above nape (fig. 4-5) • Backcomb, spray and hairnet (fig. 6-8) • Mold into a long cigar shape and pin (fig. 9-11) • Create sleek finish with straightening irons and brush (fig. 12-14) • Treat with product to give shine (fig. 15-16) • Tuck sides under base and pin into nape (fig. 17-18) • Twist remaining hair together, tuck under and pin into base (fig. 19-22) • Finish with ribbon (fig. 25-26)

 • Gel/Mousse in das Haar geben und gerade fönen (Abb. 1-3) • Haare hinten abteilen und Haare über dem Nacken zum Pferdeschwanz binden (Abb. 4-5) • Toupieren, Haarspray aufsprühen und Haarnetz aufsetzen (Abb. 6-8) • Zigarrenförmig stylen und feststecken (Abb. 9-11) • Mit Glätteisen und Bürste einen eleganten Look kreieren (Abb. 12-14) • Gel/Mousse in das Haar geben, damit es glänzt (Abb. 15-16) • Das Seitenhaar unter das Deckhaar schieben und am Nacken feststecken (Abb. 17-18) • Das übrige Haar zu einem Schwanz verdrehen, unter das Deckhaar schieben und feststecken (Abb. 19-22) • Mit einem Band verzieren (Abb. 25-26)

 • Applicare il prodotto e allisciare con il phon (figure 1-3) • Dividere la zona posteriore e fare una coda sulla nuca (figure 4-5) • Cotonare spruzzare e coprire con una retina (figure 6-8) • Arrotolare e fermare (figure 9-11) • Allisciare con la piastra e la spazzola (figure 12-14) • Applicare il prodotto per dare lucentezza (figure 15-16) • Portare i lati sotto la base e fermare sulla nuca (17-18) • Attorcigliare i capelli rimanenti, portandoli sotto la base e fermare (figure 19-22) • Decorare con un nastro (figure 25-26)

 • Traitez au produit et séchez au séchoir pour raidir les cheveux (fig. 1-3) • Séparez la section arrière et placez la queue de cheval au-dessus de la nuque (fig. 4-5) • Peignez en arrière, vaporisez et mettez sous filet à cheveux (fig. 6-8) • Moulez en forme de long cigare et épinglez (fig. 9-11) • Créez une finition élégante avec des fers à raidir et brossez (fig. 12-14) • Traitez au produit pour donner du brillant (fig. 15-16) • Placez les côtés sous la base et maintenez à l'aide d'une épingle sur la nuque (fig. 17-18) • Enroulez ensemble le reste des cheveux, glissez-les en dessous et épinglez dans la base (fig. 19-22) • Finissez avec un ruban (fig. 25-26)

 • Tratar el cabello con producto y secar para alisar. (Fig. 1-3) • Dividir la parte posterior y hacer una cola sobre la nuca. (Fig. 4-5) • Peinar hacia atrás, rociar con laca y colocar el postizo. (Fig. 6-8) • Moldear en la forma de un largo puro habano y sujetar con clips. (Fig. 9-11) • Crear un acabado elegante con un cepillo y una plancha de alisar. (Fig. 12-14) • Aplicar producto para dar brillo. (Fig. 15-16) • Colocar las partes laterales bajo la baje y sujetar con clips a la nuca. (Fig. 17-18) • Enrollar el cabello restante junto, colocar por debajo y sujetar con clips a la base. (Fig. 19-22) • Acabar con un lazo. (Fig. 25-26)

 •トリートメント剤で整え、ブローしてまっすぐにする。（図1-3）•バックをセクション分けして、えりあしの上でポニーテールを作る。（図4-5）•バックコームをして逆毛を立てる。スプレーをかけヘアネットで覆う。（図6-8）•長い葉巻の形を作り、ピンで留める（図9-11）•ストレートアイロンを用いて、なめらかさを出す。ブラッシングをする。（図12-14）•トリートメント剤でつやをだす。（図15-16）•サイドをベースの下にしまいこみ、えりあしにピンで留める。（図17-18）•残りのヘアを一緒にツイストして下にしまいこみ、ベースの中にピンで留める。（図19-22）• リボンで仕上げる。（図25-26）

 •头发用发剂处理，吹直(图1-3) •分离后发，在后颈扎成马尾(图4-5) •逆梳，喷胶，加发罩(图6-8) •定型成长雪筒状，夹住(图9-11) •用直发器和梳子做润滑效果(图12-14) •用发剂处理取光滑效果(图15-16) •将边发塞入发基，夹在后颈(图17-18) •编其余的头发，塞入并夹在发基(图19-22) •用发带定型(图25-26)

 • ضع منتج التصفيف على الشعر ونشفه بالهواء الساخن لتمليسه (الصور ١ الى ٣) • أفصل الجزء الخلفي عن بقية الشعر وأربطه على شكل ذيل الفرس فوق قفا العنق (الصورتين ٤ و٥) • مشّط ذيل الفرس بالإتجاه المعاكس ثم رشه عليه وضع عليه شبكة شعر (الصور ٦ الى ٨) • صفف ذيل الفرس الآن على شكل أنبوب مستطيل وثبته بدبابيس (الصور ٩ الى ١١) • ملّس بقية الشعر بواسطة ملقط مسخّن كهربائياً مع تسريحه بالفرشاة لإضفاء مظهر منسدل (الصور ١٢ الى ١٤) • ضع منتج يعطي لمعاناً للشعر (الصورتين ١٥ و١٦) • إفتل الجوانب تحت القاعدة وثبتها بدبابيس (الصورتين ١٧ و١٨) • إفتل الشعر الباقي سوياً وأبرمه نحو الداخل مع تثبيته بالدبابيس الى القاعدة (الصور ١٩ الى ٢٢) • وأخيراً ضع الشريط حول الشعر للزينة (الصورتين ٢٥ و١٦)

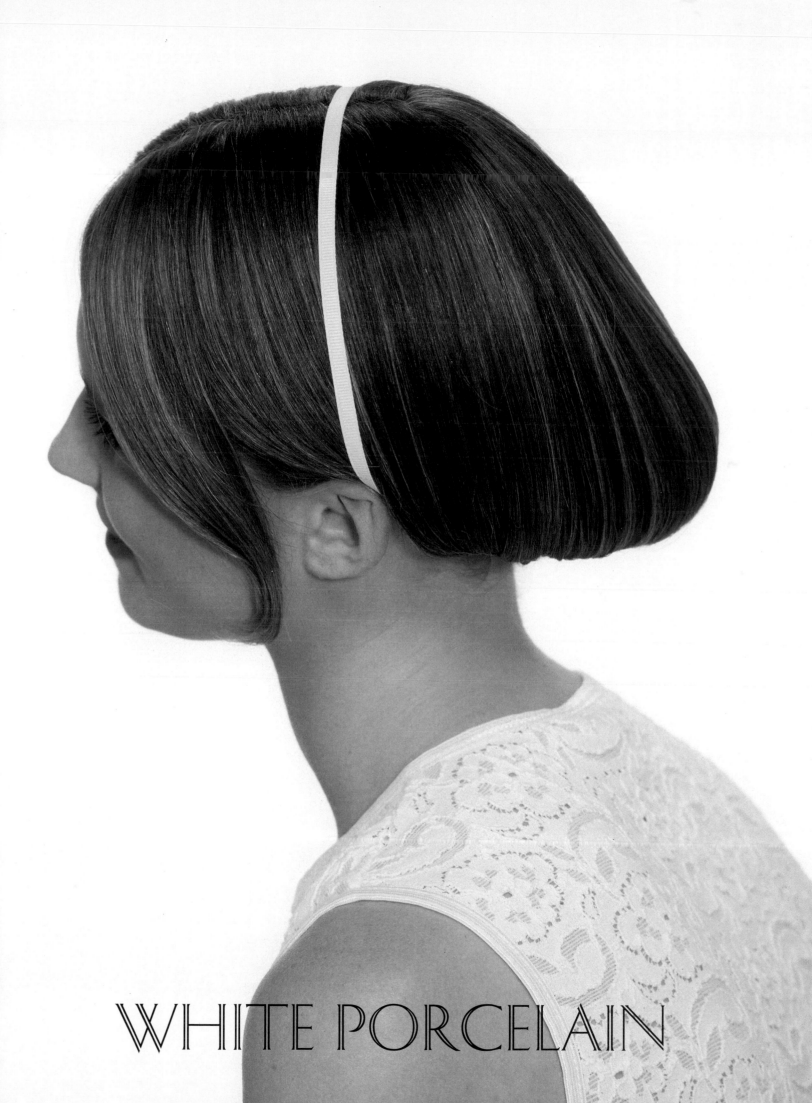

WHITE PORCELAIN

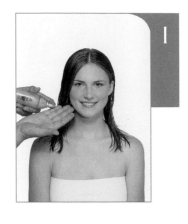

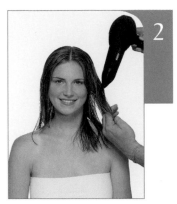

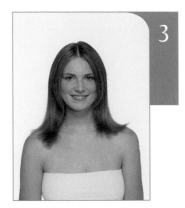

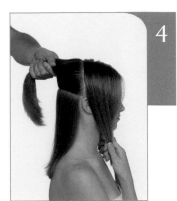

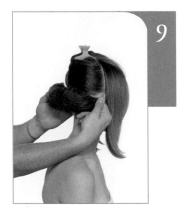

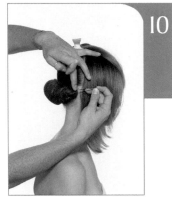

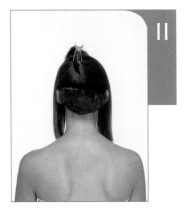

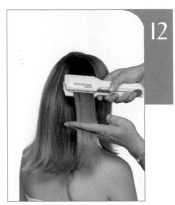

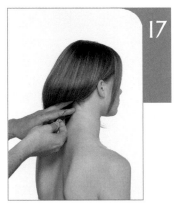

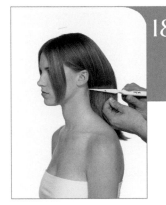

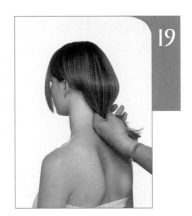

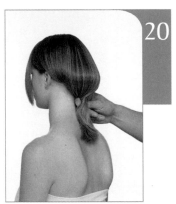

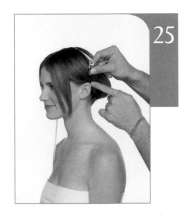

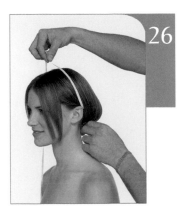

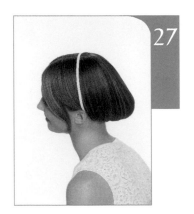

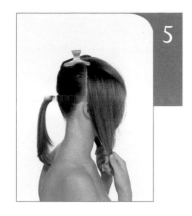

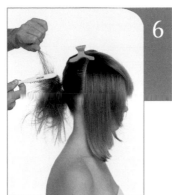

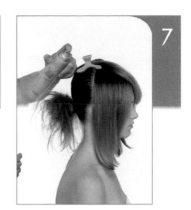

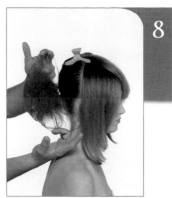

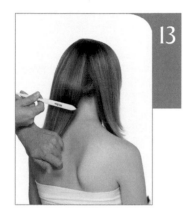

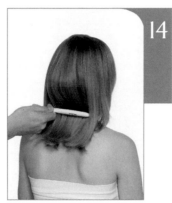

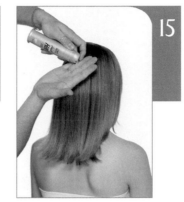

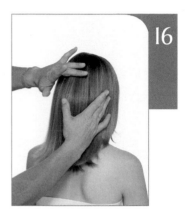

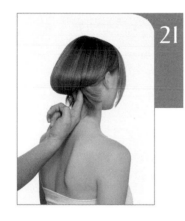

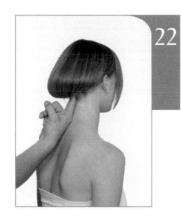

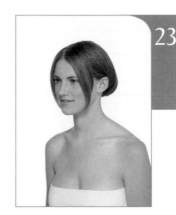

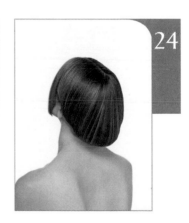

WHITE LIGHTNING

• Treat with product and blow-dry with diffuser to create soft curls (fig. 2-6) • Section a circle of 8cm diameter around crown. Place ponytail below crown (fig. 7) • Place hair band halfway down ponytail, roll forward and pin to create base on crown (fig. 8-10) • Twist back area up and pin onto base (fig. 11-13) • Divide front area into three. Pin sides and most of front into base (fig. 14-17) • Take small strands from front and pin into base creating criss-cross pattern (fig. 18-22)

• Gel/Mousse in das Haar geben und mit Diffusor fönen, damit sich die Locken weich kringeln (Abb. 2-6) • Einen runden Haarabschnitt von 8 cm Durchmesser um den Scheitel herum abtrennen. Den Pferdeschwanz unter dem Scheitel positionieren (Abb. 7) • Das Haarband auf halber Länge des Pferdeschwanzes befestigen, Pferdeschwanz nach vorne rollen und am Scheitel feststecken (Abb. 8-10) • Das Nackenhaar nach oben drehen und am Unterhaar feststecken (Abb. 11-13) • Haare dreiteilen. Die Seiten und die meisten Haare vorne am Unterhaar feststecken (Abb. 14-17) • Kleine Strähnchen aus dem Gesichtsbereich am Unterhaar feststecken, bis ein Kreuzmuster entsteht (Abb. 18-22)

• Applicare il prodotto e asciugare con il diffusore per creare dei riccioli morbidi (figure 2-6) • Dividere una sezione circolare di 8cm di diametro sulla sommita' del capo e fare una coda (figura 7) • Mettere un elastico a meta' coda e avvolgere in avanti e fermare per creare la base (figure 8-10) • Attorcigliare e fermare sulla base (figure 11-13) • Dividere in tre parti. Fermare i lati e la maggior parte della zona anteriore sulla base (figure 14-17) • Prendere delle piccole ciocche dalla parte anteriore e fermarle sulla base creando un motivo incrociato (figure 18-22)

• Traitez au produit et séchez au séchoir avec un diffuseur pour créer des mèches douces (fig. 2-6) • Séparez un cercle de 8 cm de diamètre sur le haut de la tête. Placez la queue de cheval sous le haut de la tête (fig. 7) • Placez le bandeau au milieu de la queue de cheval, roulez vers l'avant et maintenez à l'aide d'une épingle pour créer une base sur le haut de la tête (fig. 8-10) • Réenroulez la section vers le haut et épinglez dans la base (fig. 11-13) • Divisez en trois. Epinglez les côtés et la plus grande partie du devant dans la base (fig. 14-17) • Prenez de petites mèches sur le devant et épinglez dans la base pour créer un motif entrecroisé (fig. 18-22)

• Aplicar producto y secar con un difusor para crear rizos suaves. (Fig. 2-6) • Separar un círculo de 8 cm de diámetro alrededor de la coronilla. Hacer la cola por debajo de la coronilla. (Fig. 7) • Colocar una goma a la mitad de la cola, enrollar hacia delante y sujetar con clips para crear la base en la coronilla. (Fig. 8-10) • Enrollar la parte posterior y sujetar con clips a la base. (Fig. 11-13) • Dividir en tres partes. Sujetar con clips las partes laterales y la mayor parte de la sección frontal a la base. (Fig. 14-17) • Tomar pequeñas hebras de la parte delantera y sujetar con clips a la base creando un dibujo entrelazado. (Fig. 18-22)

•トリートメント剤で整える。ディフューザーを用いてブローし、ソフトなカールを作る。(図2-6) •クラウンの周りに直径8cmの円形のセクションを作る。クラウンの下でポニーテールを作る。(図7) •ポニーテールの途中真ん中にヘアバンドを使い、前方へ巻き、ピンで留めてクラウンの上にベースを作る。(図8-10) •バックを上に向けてツイストし、ベースにピンで留める。(図11-13) •3つのセクションに分ける。サイドとフロントの大部分をベースにピンで留める。(図14-17) •フロントから小さい束をとり、ベースにピンで留め、十字模様を作る。(図18-22)

•用发剂处理头发，吹干形成卷曲(图2-6) •头顶出取直径8厘米的一片头发。头顶下扎成马尾(图7) •马尾半中扎发带，向前卷，夹住以形成头顶发基(图8-10) •向上编结后发，夹入发基(图11-13) •发分三份，夹边发和最前面的头发入发基(图14-17) •取前发的小发缕，夹入发基，形成十字图案(图18-22)

• ضع منتج التصفيف على الشعر ونشفه بجهاز التشيف بالهواء الساخن المزود بفوهة ناشرة لتكوين تجاعيد ناعمة (الصور ٢ الى ٦) • أفصل دائرة قطرها ٨ سم حول ذروة الرأس وأربطها على شكل ذيل الفرس واتركها على ذروة الرأس (الصورة ٧) • ضع حلقة الربط على منتصف ذيل الفرس ولف القسم العلوي من الذيل نحو الأمام مع تثبيته بدبابيس لتكوين قاعدة على ذروة الرأس (الصور ٨ الى ١٠) • إفتل الشعر الخلفي نحو أعلى وثبته بدبابيس الى القاعدة (الصور ١١ الى ١٣) • إقسم الى ثلاثة أقسام ثم ثبت الجوانب واغلب الجزء الأمامي الى القاعدة (الصور ١٤ الى ١٧) • إلتقط خصل صغيرة من الأمام وثبتها الى القاعدة بدبابيس لخلق نمط متشابك (الصور ١٨ الى ٢٢)

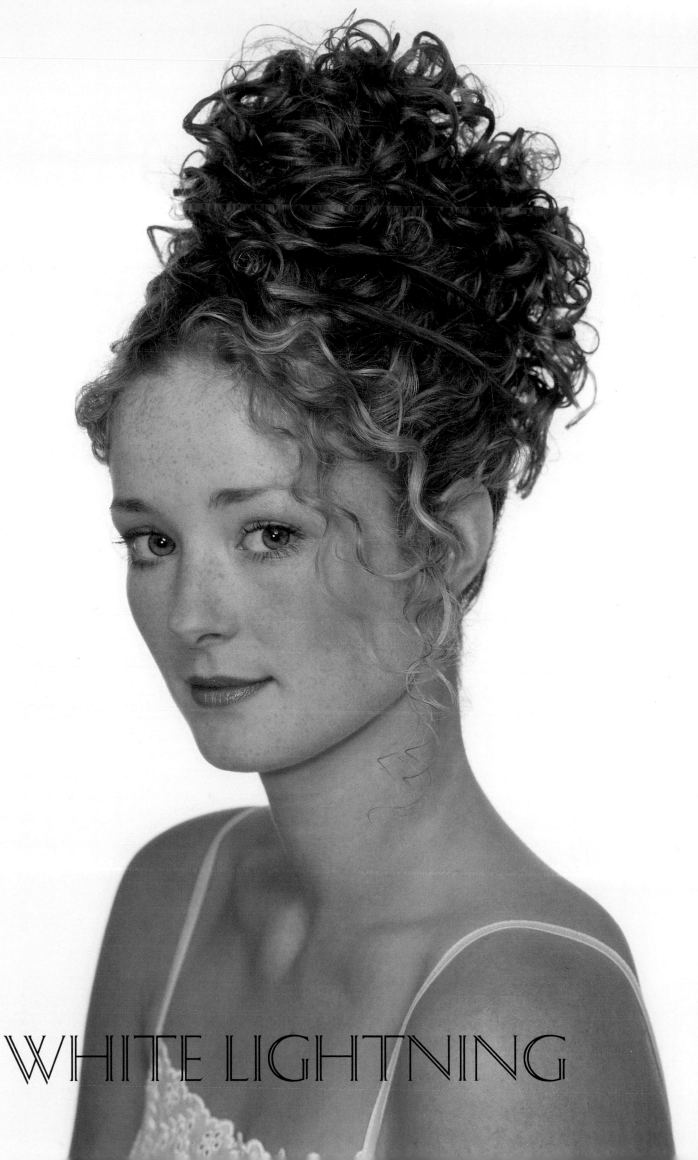

WHITE LIGHTNING

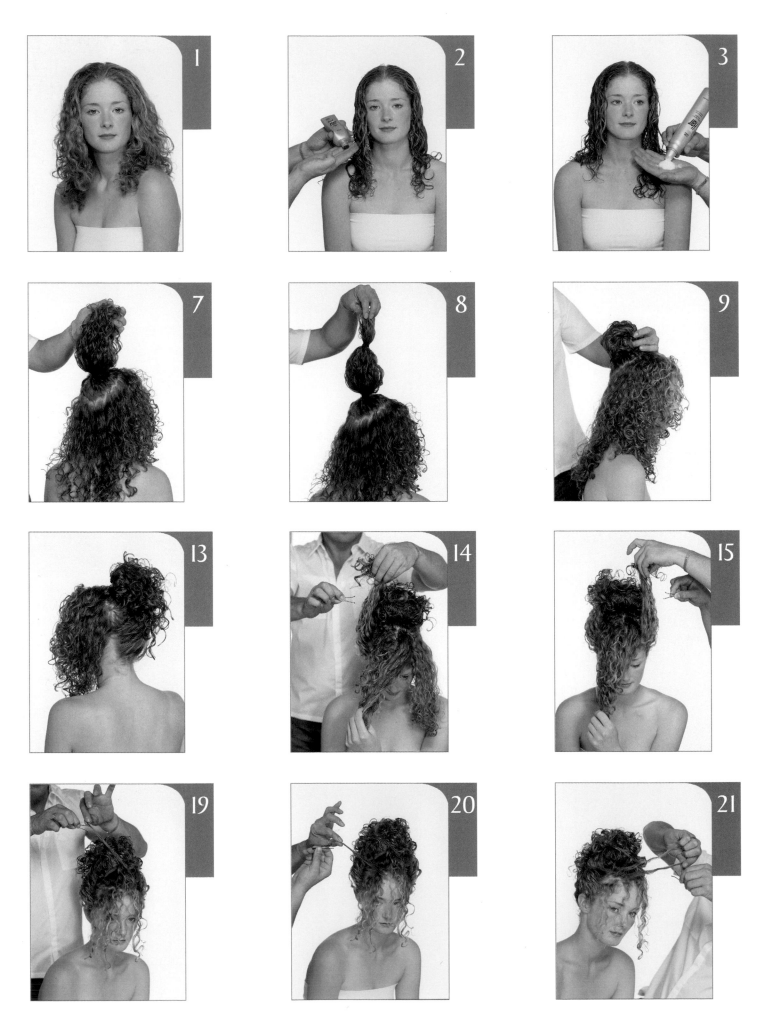

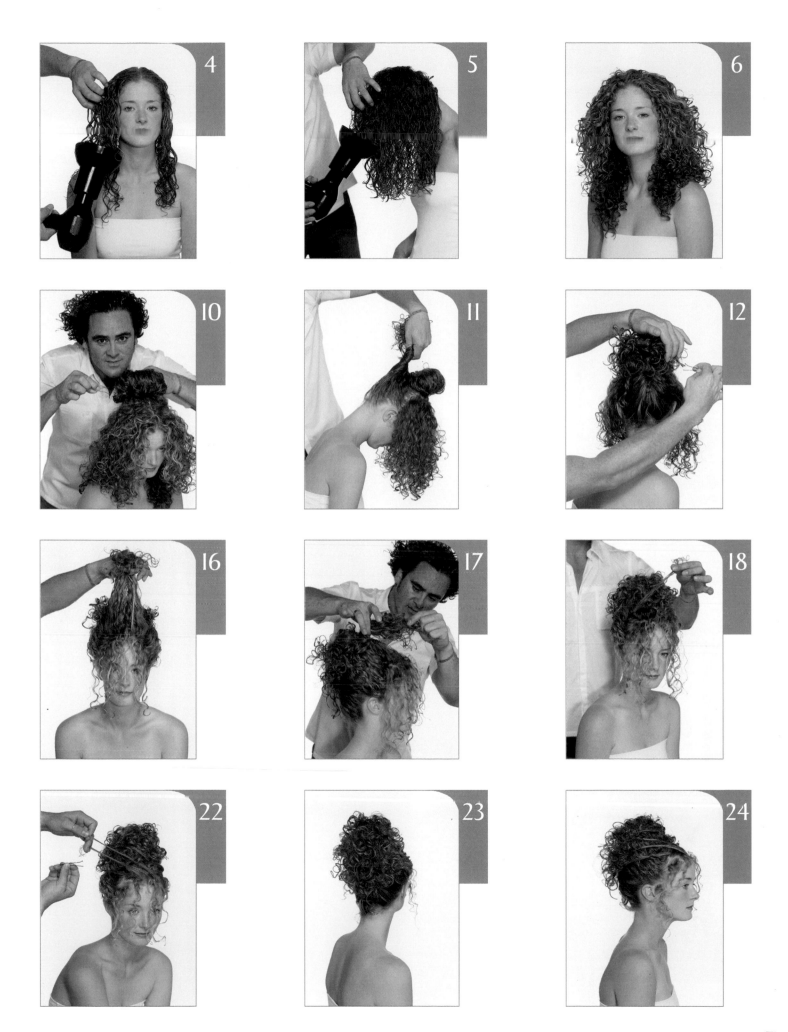

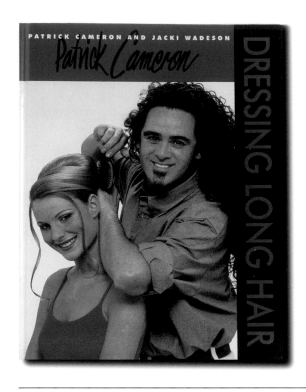

Patrick Cameron: Dressing Long Hair

Patrick's first book is a timeless classic. Featuring over 30 different long hair designs and techniques.

- A magical mix of twists, weaves, curls and braids.

- Over 450 full colour photographs.

- Detailed instructions and professional tips on styling and dressing long hair.

Patrick Cameron: Dressing Long Hair Book 2

- 15 step by step long hair styles.

- Hundreds of detailed step by step photographs.

- Imaginative format of fold out pages to view at a glance.

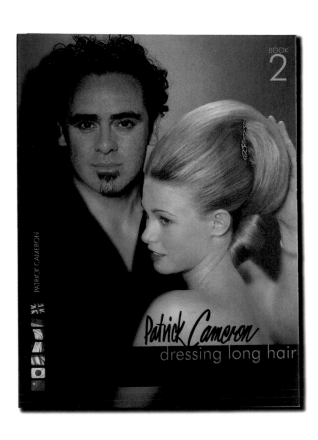

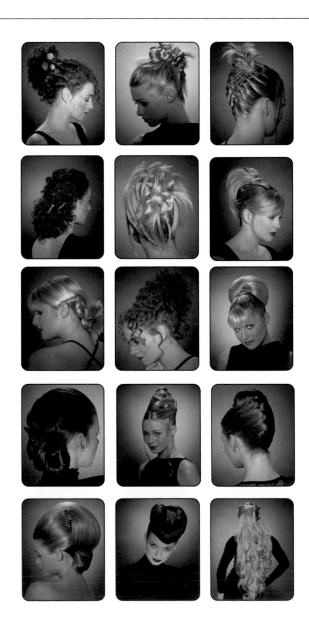

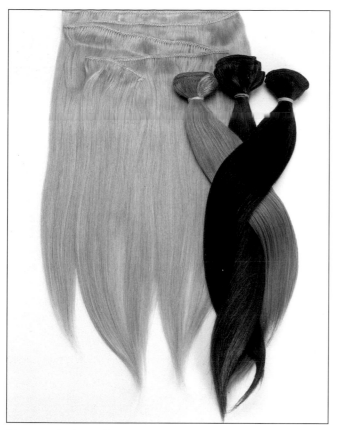

Human hair wefts

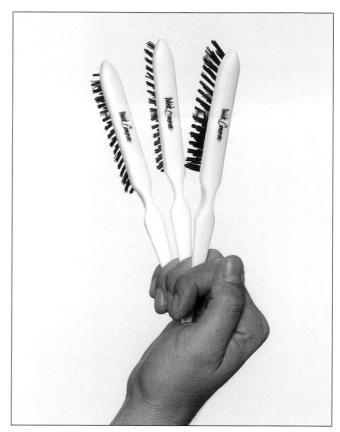

Long hair styling brush

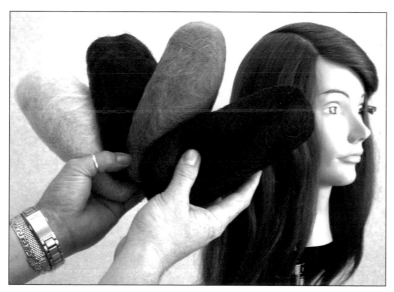

Synthetic hair padding

All merchandise is available from:

Marco Everard
Patrick Cameron Hair International
30 Aden Grove
London N16 9NJ
United Kingdom

Tel/Fax: +44 (0) 20 7923 0599
e-mail: marco@patrick-cameron.com
www.patrick-cameron.com

VIDEOS

VIDEO 1

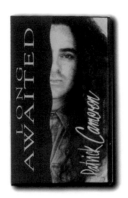

"Long Awaited"
Running time approx.
45 minutes.

Six long hair designs
from Patrick's
European collection.

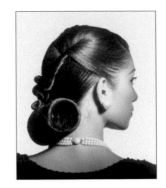

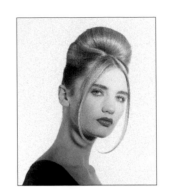

VIDEO 2

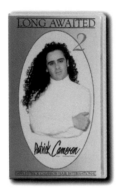

"Long Awaited 2"
Running time approx.
60 minutes.

Six more long hair
looks from Patrick's
Royal collection.

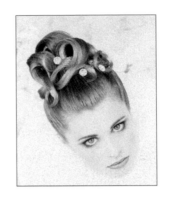

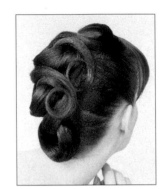

VIDEO 3

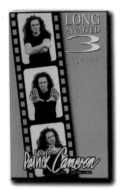

"Long Awaited 3"
Running time approx.
45 minutes.

Six new styles to give
you that extra edge in
the fashion stakes of
dressing long hair.

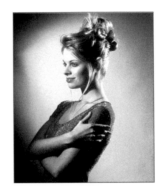

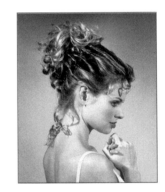

VIDEO 4

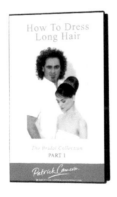

**"The Bridal
Collection: Part 1"**
Running time approx.
45 minutes.

Classic long hair
techniques and
contemporary styling
create the perfect bridal
video.

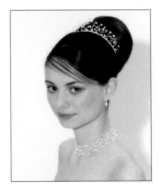

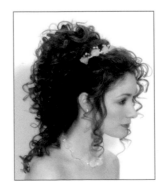

VIDEO 5

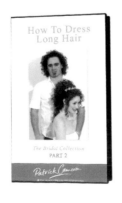

**"The Bridal
Collection: Part 2"**
Running time approx.
45 minutes.

Six more beautiful step
by step bridal styles.

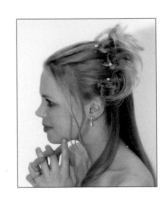

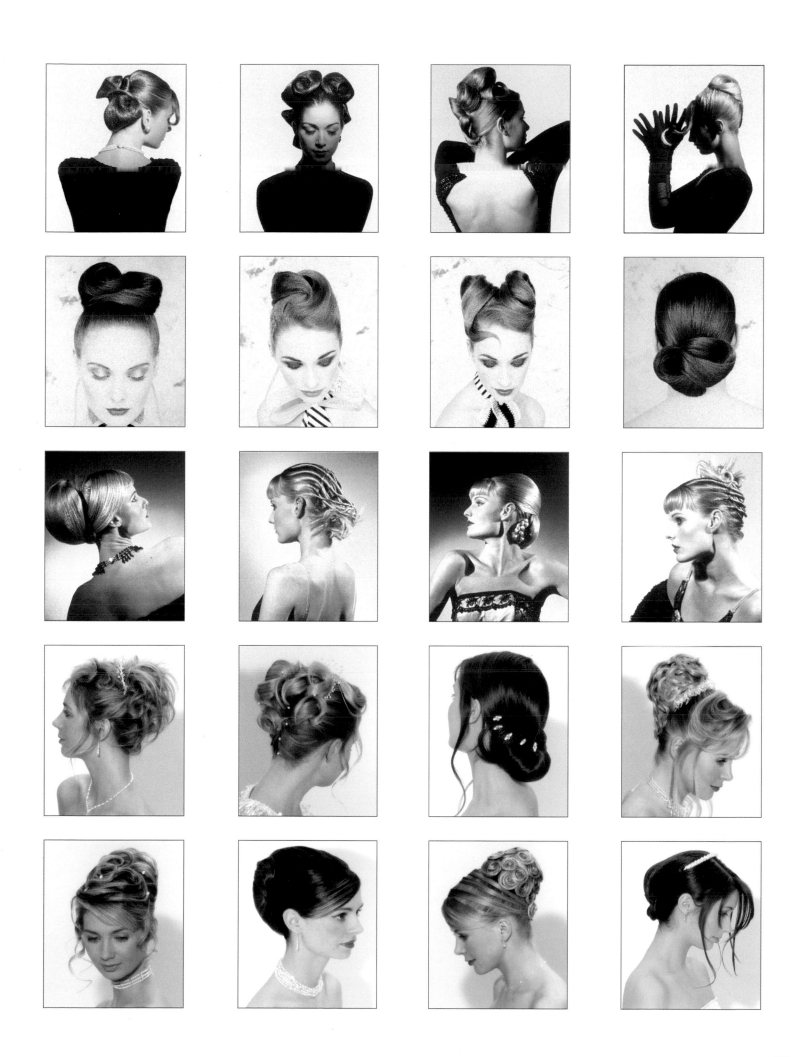

In 1997 Patrick Cameron opened his own training school to give students intensive tuition in the art of dressing long hair. Courses take place in London and around the world on a regular basis under Patrick's personal guidance and supervision.
"I like to teach students just one or two steps at a time to break down the style into a logical, easy to understand structure" says Patrick. "Usually we cover at least four styles a day and the results, using this method with small groups of students is superb. My students have ranged from newly qualified hairdressers keen to come to grips with long hair, to experienced professionals looking for further inspiration. The exclusive nature of this course allows me to concentrate on each persons individual needs."

1997 eröffnete Patrick Cameron seine eigene Friseurschule, in der er seinen Studenten und Studentinnen die Frisierkunst an langem Haar zeigt. Die Kurse finden regelmäßig in London und rund um den Globus unter Patricks persönlicher Führung und Aufsicht statt.
„Ich zeige meinen Studenten jeweils nur ein, zwei Schritte, damit sie die logische, leicht verständliche Struktur der Frisur begreifen", so Patrick. „Normalerweise bringen wir unseren Studenten mindestens vier verschiedene Frisuren pro Tag bei. Glauben Sie mir, mit dieser Methode mit kleinen Studiengruppen lassen sich die Ergebnisse wirklich sehen! Zu mir kommen Friseure, die ihren Abschluss gerade erst in der Tasche haben und wissen möchten, wie sie am besten mit langen Haaren umgehen, aber auch Friseure mit langjähriger Erfahrung, die neue Anregungen suchen. Der Kurs ist so aufgebaut, dass ich mich ganz nach den Wünschen der einzelnen Teilnehmer richten kann.

Nel 1997 Patrick Cameron decise di aprire una scuola dedicata esclusivamente all'arte della acconciatura raccolta. I corsi si tengono a Londra dove Patrick risiede e a volte in trasferta in altri paesi del mondo sempre sotto la guida e supervisione personale di Patrick.
Mi piace dimostrare agli studenti uno o due passaggi alla volta per spiegare il look in modo logico e facile da comprendere, dice Patrick. Di solito realizziamo un minimo di quattro stili al giorno, e i risultati quando si ha un numero ridotto di studenti sono straordinari. Fra i partecipanti ci sono sia parrucchieri appena qualificati che desiderano lavorare con i capelli lunghi che professionisti esperti alla ricerca di nuove idee. La natura esclusiva di questo corso mi consente di concentrarmi sulle esigenze di ogni persona.

En 1997, Patrick Cameron a ouvert son centre de formation pour fournir à ses élèves une éducation intensive dans l'art de coiffer les cheveux longs. Les stages ont lieu à Londres et un peu partout dans le monde à intervalles réguliers sous la direction et la surveillance personnelle de Patrick.
'J'aime n'enseigner à mes étudiants qu'une seule ou deux étapes à la fois afin de décomposer la procédure de création de style en une structure logique et facile à comprendre' déclare Patrick. 'Nous traitons généralement environ au moins quatre styles par jour et les résultats obtenus par cette méthode avec de petits groupes d'étudiants sont superbes. Mes étudiants vont des coiffeurs nouvellement formés désireux de maîtriser les techniques de coiffure des cheveux longs, aux professionnels expérimentés à la recherche d'un supplément d'inspiration. La nature exclusive de ce stage me permet de me concentrer sur les besoins individuels de chacun des stagiaires.'

En 1997 Patrick Cameron abrió su propia escuela para ofrecer a los estudiantes formación intensiva en el arte de peinar el cabello largo. Los cursos tienen lugar en Londres y en otras partes del mundo con regularidad bajo la supervisión y el asesoramiento personal de Patrick.
"Me gusta enseñar a los alumnos uno o dos pasos a la vez, para desglosar el peinado en una estructura lógica y fácil de comprender", explica Patrick. "Normalmente cubrimos como mínimo cuatro peinados al día, y los resultados de utilizar este método con grupos reducidos de estudiantes son excelentes. Entre mis alumnos se cuentan desde peluqueros que acaban de obtener el título, ansiosos por aprender a tratar el pelo largo, hasta profesionales expertos que buscan nueva inspiración. La naturaleza exclusiva de este curso me permite concentrarme en las necesidades individuales de cada persona.

1997年、パトリック・キャメロンはロングヘアのドレッシングを徹底訓練するためのトレーニングスクールを開校しました。以来、パトリック自らの指導と指揮のもと、ロンドンをはじめ世界中で定期的にコースを開講しています。「私のスクールではスタイルを細かく分けて一度につきワン・ステップかツー・ステップずつ、論理的にわかりやすく系統立てて教えるようにしています。小人数のグループ制をとり、通常、1日あたり4つ以上のスタイルをお教えしてすばらしい効果をあげています。生徒の皆さんはロングヘアの扱い方をしっかり身につけたいという美容師の資格を取得したばかりの方たちから、インスピレーションを求める経験豊富なプロの皆さんまでいろいろです。私が直接、生徒さんの個人個人のニーズに十分にお応えするようにしている点がスクールの特徴です」とパトリックは語ります。

帕奇克·卡迈龙1997年创立了他自己的培训学校。在长发发饰艺术上，给学生以精心指导。帕奇克定期在伦敦和世界各地亲临指导授课。
帕奇克说：“我喜欢教学生一次一两步骤，把发型分解成有逻辑的、简单易懂的结构。通常我们一天至少教四个发型，并且在小班组里，这种方法效果非常良好。我的学生有学习长发发饰，刚从事美发行业的新秀，也有来寻求灵感的资深专家。课程的特色是专注于每个学生的需要。”

في عام ١٩٩٧ افتتح باتريك كاميرون مدرسة تدريب خاصة به لتوفير تدريب مكثّف الى الطلاب في فن تسريح وتصفيف الشعر الطويل. تجري دورات هذا المعهد في لندن كما في أنحاء أخرى حول العالم على أساس منتظم تحت إشراف وتوجيه السيد باتريك بنفسه. يقول باتريك: «إنني أعلم تلامذتي بطريقة متدرجة، ليس أكثر من خطوة أو خطوتين في كل مرة، لكي أتمكن من تجزئة التسريحة إلى خطوات متسلسلة منطقية يسهل فهمها. إننا ننفّذ عادة أربع تسريحات في اليوم الواحد بتطبيق هذا الأسلوب مع مجموعات صغيرة من الطلاب مما يوفر لنا نتائج ممتازة. أما تلامذتي فمنهم من تخرّج حديثاً ويرغب في التدرب على أساليب تصفيف الشعر الطويل ومنهم من هو ممارس متمهّن ينشد أفكاراً وآراءً جديدة. إن المنهج المتبع في دورات التدريب هذه يساعدني على التركيز على الإحتياجات الشخصية لكل طالب.

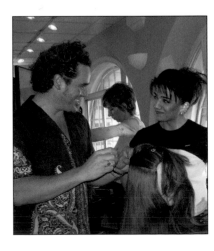

For further information on the
Patrick Cameron training school
please visit our website at
www.patrick-cameron.com
or contact Studio Manager:
Marco Everard
Patrick Cameron Seminars,
30 Aden Grove, London N16 9NJ
United Kingdom

Tel/Fax: +44 (0) 20 7923 0599
e-mail: marco@patrick-cameron.com

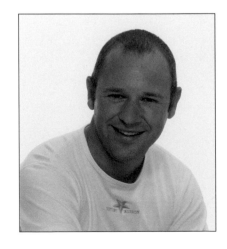

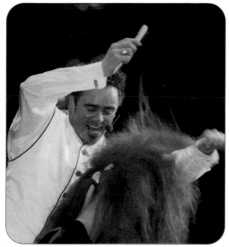

P atrick Cameron has justly earned his place in hairdressing's hall of fame as one of the world's leading platform artists, giving him the title, 'The Maestro of Long Hair.'

A regular on television screens both in the UK and overseas and appearing at the most prestigious global hairdressing events all over the world, Patrick continues to educate and inspire many with his visual and often avant garde stage productions. Using his skills gained whilst working as a salon stylist and platform artist, he combines the commercial aspects of speed required for salon work with the theatrical, a combination that enthralls his audiences.

Taking his inspiration from an eclectic variety of sources, Patrick has year after year grabbed the hairdressing headlines when presenting his innovative collections.

In addition to his global appearances and London based Training School, Patrick always takes time out of his busy schedule to visit at least 5 UK colleges each year where he will present Look and Learn seminars to eager young students, many of whom otherwise would not get a chance to see him demonstrate and present his many talents.

Patrick's philosophy is one that has taken him around the world many times and it is one that translates well into any language – "My aim is to create natural looks that make women feel feminine," says Patrick. "When I am presenting on stage I try to break down my techniques into simple step by step instructions so that my audiences can go away and think I can do that. If they leave the show feeling like that, then I have done my job."

Patrick's zest, energy, vitality and dedication to his craft seem never ending. One of the most charming and talented people you could ever meet, Patrick has justly earned his title, 'The Maestro of Long Hair'.

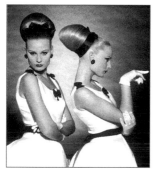

"Breakfast at Tiffany's" 1996

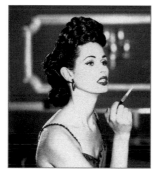

"Tango" 1997

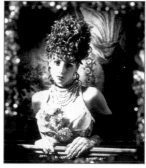

"Opera" 1998

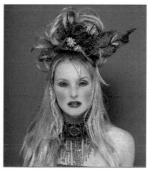

"Global Tribe" 1999

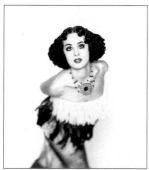

"Arts and Crafts" 2000

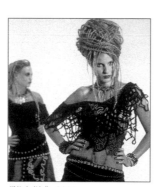

"Nightlife" 2001

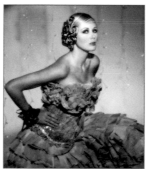

"Visionaire" 2002

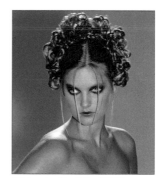

"Bohemian Revolution" 2003

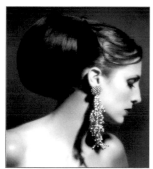

"Provocateur" 2004

For further information about Patrick Cameron International
please contact his business partner
Susan Callaghan
Patrick Cameron Hair International
PO Box 124 Chester, Cheshire CH1 6ZF

Tel: 01244 880807 fax: 01244 881140
email: sue@patrick-cameron.com

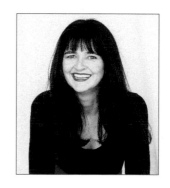

ACKNOWLEDGMENTS

Hair:

PATRICK CAMERON

Photography:

Alistair Hughes

Make-up and clothes styling:

Alison Chesterton

Hair styling products:

Wella

Models:

Boss Models Manchester

Nemesis Models Manchester

Designed by:

Umbrella Communications

With thanks to:

Marco Everard

Sue Callaghan

Alison Chesterton

Marco Erbi

Terry Fisher

Paul Jones

Will White

Maureen Barrymore

Phil Ollerenshaw

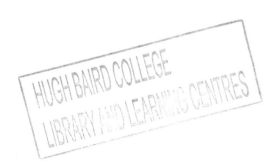

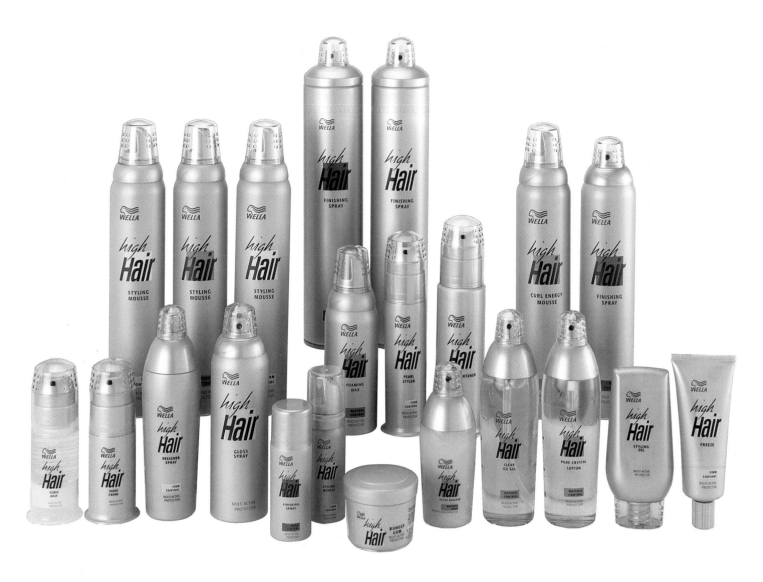

"Give shape to your ideas. From classical finish to the latest styles, it's easy with High Hair."

High Hair is a salon exclusive brand.

Wella (UK) Limited
Wella Road,
Basingstoke,
RG22 4AF
United Kingdom

Tel: +44 (0) 1256 320 202
Fax: + 44(0) 1256 471 518

Wella AG
Berliner Allee 65,
64274 Darmstadt,
Germany

Tel: +49 (0) 6151 340
Fax: +49 (0) 6151 342 080

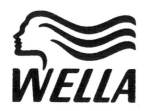

First published 2001 by
PATRICK CAMERON HAIR INTERNATIONAL
30 Aden Grove,
London N16 9NJ
United Kingdom

ISBN 0-9541106-0-9

Printed in Great Britain by
L&S Printing Ltd, Worthing, West Sussex.

Colour reproduction by
Ocean Colour Ltd.

Designed by
Umbrella Communications Ltd.